Collaborative Partnerships to Advance Practice

Editors

SUZIE C. NELSON
JESSICA K. JEFFREY
MARK S. BORER
BARRY D. SARVET

CHILD AND ADOLESCENT PSYCHIATRIC CLINICS OF NORTH AMERICA

www.childpsych.theclinics.com

Consulting Editor
TODD E. PETERS

October 2021 • Volume 30 • Number 4

ELSEVIER

1600 John F. Kennedy Boulevard • Suite 1800 • Philadelphia, Pennsylvania, 19103-2899

http://www.theclinics.com

**CHILD AND ADOLESCENT PSYCHIATRIC CLINICS OF NORTH AMERICA Volume 30, Number 4
October 2021 ISSN 1056–4993, ISBN-13: 978-0-323-84870-1**

Editor: Lauren Boyle
Developmental Editor: Arlene Campos

Child and Adolescent Psychiatric Clinics of North America (ISSN 1056-4993) is published quarterly by Elsevier Inc., 360 Park Avenue South, New York, NY 10010-1710. Months of issue are January, April, July, and October. Business and Editorial Offices: 1600 John F. Kennedy Boulevard, Suite 1800, Philadelphia, PA 19103-2899. Periodicals postage paid at New York, NY and additional mailing offices. Subscription prices are $348.00 per year (US individuals), $844.00 per year (US institutions), $100.00 per year (US & Canadian students), $388.00 per year (Canadian individuals), $899.00 per year (Canadian institutions), $446.00 per year (international individuals), $899.00 per year (international institutions), and $200.00 per year (international students). International air speed delivery is included in all *Clinics* subscription prices. All prices are subject to change without notice. **POSTMASTER:** Send address changes to *Child and Adolescent Psychiatric Clinics of North America*, Elsevier Health Sciences Division, Subscription Customer Service, 3251 Riverport Lane, Maryland Heights, MO 63043. **Customer Service: 1-800-654-2452 (U.S. and Canada); 314-447-8871 (outside U.S. and Canada). Fax: 314-447-8029. E-mail:** JournalsCustomerService-usa@elsevier.com **(for print support) or** journalsonlinesupport-usa@elsevier.com **(for online support).**

Reprints. For copies of 100 or more of articles in this publication, please contact the Commercial Reprints Department, Elsevier Inc., 360 Park Avenue South, New York, New York 10010-1710 Tel.: 212-633-3874; Fax: 212-633-3820, E-mail: reprints@elsevier.com.

Child and Adolescent Psychiatric Clinics of North America is covered in *MEDLINE/PubMed (Index Medicus)*, *ISI, SSCI, Research Alert, Social Search, Current Contents,* and *EMBASE/Excerpta Medica.*

Contributors

CONSULTING EDITOR

TODD E. PETERS, MD, FAPA
Vice President/Chief Medical Officer (CMO), Chief Medical Information Officer (CMIO), Sheppard Pratt Health System, Baltimore, Maryland

EDITORS

SUZIE C. NELSON, MD, DFAACAP, FAPA
Assistant Professor, Associate Program Director Child and Adolescent Psychiatry Fellowship, Wright State University Boonshoft School of Medicine, Department of Psychiatry, Dayton, Ohio

JESSICA K. JEFFREY, MD, MPH, MBA, FAPA, DF-AACAP
Associate Professor of Psychiatry, Associate Medical Director of Ambulatory Operations, Associate Director, Lead Psychiatrist, UCLA Department of Psychiatry and Biobehavioral Sciences, Division of Population Behavioral Health, Division of Child and Adolescent Psychiatry, UCLA Behavioral Health Associates, UCLA Semel Institute of Neuroscience and Human Behavior, Los Angeles, California

MARK S. BORER, MD, DLFAPA, DLFAACAP
Child and Adolescent Psychiatrist, Owner and President, Psychiatric Access for Central Delaware, P.A. Board Certified Child and Adolescent, General Adult Psychiatry, Family Psychiatry, Dover, Delaware; Collaborative Psychiatry and Primary Care Consultation with Creatri(cs Pro-Pack Toolkit®, Delaware Child Psychiatry Access Program (DCPAP) for Primary Care Professionals, Delegate for Delaware to American Academy of Child and Adolescent Psychiatry, Co-chair AACAP's Healthcare Access and Economics Committee

BARRY D. SARVET, MD, FAACAP, DFAPA
Professor and Chair, Department of Psychiatry, University of Massachusetts Medical School-Baystate, Baystate Medical Center, Springfield, Massachusetts

AUTHORS

MARK S. BORER, MD, DLFAPA, DLFAACAP
Child and Adolescent Psychiatrist, Owner and President, Psychiatric Access for Central Delaware, P.A. Board Certified Child and Adolescent, General Adult Psychiatry, Family Psychiatry, Dover, Delaware; Collaborative Psychiatry and Primary Care Consultation with Creatri(cs Pro-Pack Toolkit®, Delaware Child Psychiatry Access Program (DCPAP) for Primary Care Professionals, Delegate for Delaware to American Academy of Child and Adolescent Psychiatry, Co-chair AACAP's Healthcare Access and Economics Committee

SUSAN H. MCDANIEL, PhD, ABPP
Dr Laurie Sands Distinguished Professor of Families and Health, Director, Institute for the Family and Chief Psychologist, Department of Psychiatry, Vice Chair, Department of Family Medicine, Director, UR Medicine Physician Faculty Communication Coaching Program, University of Rochester Medicine, Rochester New York

STEVEN CHEN, PharmD, FASHP, FCSHP, FNAP
Associate Dean for Clinical Affairs, Professor, Department of Clinical Pharmacy, University of Southern California School of Pharmacy, Los Angeles, California

WILLIAM CLARK, MD, MBA
Assistant Professor, Department of Psychiatry, Wright State University Boonshoft School of Medicine, Dayton, Ohio

PETER A. DEPERGOLA II, PhD, MTS
Department of Medicine, University of Massachusetts Medical School-Baystate, Springfield, Massachusetts; Department of Bioethics and Medical Humanities, College of Our Lady of the Elms, St. Augustine Center for Ethics, Religion, and Culture, College of Our Lady of the Elms, Chicopee, Massachusetts

JULIE A. DOPHEIDE, PharmD, BCPP, FASHP
Professor of Clinical Pharmacy, Psychiatry and the Behavioral Sciences, University of Southern California School of Pharmacy, Keck School of Medicine of USC, Los Angeles, California

GAIL A. EDELSOHN, MD, MSPH
Community Care Behavioral Health Organization, UPMC Insurance Services Division, Exton, Pennsylvania

MONA GANDHI, MSN, APRN
Psychiatric Mental Health Nurse Practitioner- Board Certified, Child Guidance Center of Mid-Fairfield County, 100 East Avenue, Norwalk, Connecticut

NASTASSIA J. HAJAL, PhD
Assistant Clinical Professor, Department of Psychiatry and Biobehavioral Sciences, Division of Population Behavioral Health, UCLA Semel Institute for Neuroscience and Human Behavior, Los Angeles, California

CAITLIN HAMMOND, MD, Maj, USAF, MC
Assistant Professor of Pediatrics, Uniformed Services University of the Health Sciences, Bethesda, Maryland; Wright State University, Dayton, Ohio

AMY HOISINGTON-STABILE, MD
Assistant Professor of Child and Adolescent Psychiatry- Clinical, The Ohio State University, Department of Psychiatry, Nationwide Children's Hospital, Columbus, Ohio

JESSICA K. JEFFREY, MD, MPH, MBA, FAPA, DF-AACAP
Associate Professor of Psychiatry, Associate Medical Director of Ambulatory Operations, Associate Director, Lead Psychiatrist, UCLA Department of Psychiatry and Biobehavioral Sciences, Division of Population Behavioral Health, Division of Child and Adolescent Psychiatry, UCLA Behavioral Health Associates, UCLA Semel Institute of Neuroscience and Human Behavior, Los Angeles, California

SHASHANK V. JOSHI, MD
Director of Training in Child & Adolescent Psychiatry, Director of School Mental Health Services, Lucile Packard Children's Hospital at Stanford, Stanford, California; Professor

of Psychiatry, Pediatrics, and Education, Stanford University School of Medicine, Stanford, California

VONDA KEELS-LOWE, MSN, CPN, PMHNP-BC, CNP
Department of Psychiatry, Nationwide Children's Hospital, Columbus, Ohio

MICHELLE KIGER, MD, Maj, USAF, MC
Associate Professor of Pediatrics, Uniformed Services University of the Health Sciences, Bethesda, Matyland, USA; Wright State University, Dayton, Ohio

KARA KNICKERBOCKER, DO, Capt, USAF, MC
Assistant Professor of Pediatrics, Wright State University, Dayton, Ohio

RAJEEV KRISHNA, MD, PhD
Child and Adolescent Psychiatrist, Behavioral Health, Department of Psychiatry, Nationwide Children's Hospital, Columbus, Ohio

PATRICIA LESTER, MD
Jane and Marc Nathanson Professor of Psychiatry, UCLA Department of Psychiatry and Biobehavioral Sciences, Los Angeles, California

DEBBIE H. LU, PharmD, MPH
Adjunct Professor, Touro University California, College of Pharmacy, Vallejo, California

ANDREW LUSTBADER, MD, FAAP
Associate Clinical Professor, Yale Child Study Center, Medical Director, Prospects Program, Child Guidance Center of Mid-Fairfield County, Director, The Therapeutic Center for Children and Families, Westport, Connecticut

SHANNON L. MAZUR, DO, MA
Assistant Professor, Department of Psychiatry, Yale University School of Medicine, New Haven, Connecticut; Department of Psychological Medicine, Yale New Haven Hospital, New Haven, Connecticut

KAYE MCGINTY, MD
Child and Adolescent Psychiatrist, Division of Child and Adolescent Psychiatry, Department of Psychiatry, Prisma Health, Greenville, South Carolina

MARCUS MERRIMAN MS, APRN-CNP, PHMNP-BC
Department of Psychiatry, Nationwide Children's Hospital, Columbus, Ohio

NORWEETA MILBURN, PhD
Professor-in-Residence, UCLA Department of Psychiatry and Biobehavioral Sciences, Los Angeles, California

CATHERINE MOGIL, PsyD
Associate Clinical Professor, UCLA Department of Psychiatry and Biobehavioral Sciences, Los Angeles, California

GITA MURTHY, MSW, MPH, LCSW
Executive Consultant, Los Angeles County Department of Mental Health + UCLA Strike Team, Altadena, California

SUZIE C. NELSON, MD, DFAACAP, FAPA
Assistant Professor, Associate Program Director Child and Adolescent Psychiatry Fellowship, Wright State University Boonshoft School of Medicine, Department of Psychiatry, Dayton, Ohio

JESSICA RAK, MSN, APRN
Psychiatric Mental Health Nurse Practitioner- Board Certified, Associate Medical Director, Prospects Extended Day Program, Child Guidance Center of Mid-Fairfield County, Clinical instructor Yale School of Nursing, Norwalk, Connecticut

ERIKA RYST, MD
Director of Nevada Leadership Education in Neurodevelopmental and Related Disabilities Program, Medical Director, Nevada Center for Excellence in Disabilities; Administrative Faculty, College of Education and Human Development, University of Nevada, Reno, Reno, Nevada

BARRY D. SARVET, MD, FAACAP, DFAPA
Professor and Chair, Department of Psychiatry, University of Massachusetts Medical School-Baystate, Baystate Medical Center, Springfield, Massachusetts

SOURAV SENGUPTA, MD, MPH
Assistant Professor, Departments of Psychiatry and Pediatrics, Jacobs School of Medicine, University at Buffalo, Buffalo, New York; Children's Psychiatry Clinic of Oishei Children's Hospital, Buffalo, New York

JONATHAN SHERIN, MD, PhD
Director, Los Angeles County Department of Mental Health, Los Angeles, California

MICHAEL SIERRA, MD
Child and Adolescent Psychiatrist, Division of Child and Adolescent Psychiatry, Department of Psychiatry, Prisma Health, Greenville, South Carolina

ANGELA L. VENEGAS-MURILLO, MD, MPH
Assistant Professor, Department of Pediatrics, College of Medicine, Charles R. Drew University of Medicine and Science, Clinical Instructor, Department of General Internal Medicine and Health Service Research, UCLA Health, Los Angeles, California

DRI WANG, PharmD, BCPP
Otsuka Pharmaceutical Development and Commercialization, Inc, Princeton, New Jersey

Contents

Promoting integrated care initiatives is an important approach to addressing growing gaps in access to mental health. This article presents a multidisciplinary review of essential team elements and how to optimize team performance. Fostering a collaborative team approach can produce more effective and efficient mental health care.

The significant and ongoing shortage of child and adolescent psychiatrists has limited access to mental health care in the pediatric population. In response to this problem, integrated/collaborative care models have been established. These models, as all imperfect things in medicine, have their own set of challenges. A careful ethical analysis of integrated/collaborative care models is essential to protect the social and emotional health and safety of children with mental illness. To this end, ethical assessment supports the use of integrated/collaborative care models, and recent studies have demonstrated the benefits of their implementation.

To identify elements of effective interprofessional education (IPE) within child and adolescent mental health (CAMH), we conducted a scoping literature review. A search of four databases revealed 32 studies that met inclusion criteria describing IPE interventions regarding CAMH. Studies included a range of medical, mental health, allied health, educational, and community professionals in clinical, school-based, and community-based settings. The majority of studies have focused on autism or general child mental health. Outcomes were generally positive but skewed toward attitudinal and knowledge-based measures. Practice-based interventions tended to support higher levels of educational outcomes, including behavioral, patient-level, or systems-level changes.

To effectively fulfill various roles in systems of care, a child and adolescent psychiatrist must first define "system of care" and become familiar with the child-serving systems that make up the overarching system of care. They should know what roles are currently being fulfilled by child and adolescent psychiatrists, recognize the challenges they may face while fulfilling these roles, and use this knowledge to become catalysts for system improvements. This article discusses these points in greater detail.

Early life adversity and trauma can jeopardize child and family well-being. Mitigating the effects of early adversity and trauma requires a tiered, public health approach that includes trauma-informed mental health promotion, prevention, screening, early intervention, and effective and equitable treatment across community ecosystems and service systems. This article describes the development of a partnership between a public academic (University of California at Los Angeles) and community mental health system (Los Angeles County Department of Mental Health) and provides a roadmap for core principles and actionable steps to implement coherent, comprehensive, and adaptive trauma-informed community systems of support for children.

Since the early 1900s when school-based health services were first introduced, models of school-based health have evolved toward comprehensive and integrated models that include mental health. New and innovative models of Comprehensive Mental Health Systems offer a range of prevention and intervention strategies that are delivered across collaborative systems of community and school-based mental health. Studies of school-based health services indicate positive outcomes in health, mental health, and education. Child and adolescent psychiatrists can work with schools by providing direct service, consultation, and technical assistance to increase access, improve health equity, and optimize mental health outcomes for all youth.

Pediatric primary care clinicians (PPCCs) are managing increasing mental health challenges in the children and adolescents they treat. Child and adolescent psychiatrists (CAPs) are increasingly involved in collaborative and integrated care (CIC) work that builds the knowledge and skills of PPCCs to manage mild to moderate mental health challenges for children and adolescents in primary care. CAPs who can establish good working relationships, communicate clearly and efficiently, and facilitate the care of this population will be successful in engaging our PPCC partners in CIC.

Jessica K. Jeffrey, Angela L. Venegas-Murillo, Rajeev Krishna, and Nastassia J. Hajal

Barriers to conducting standardized behavioral health screening within pediatric primary care settings include engaging youth and families, limited time available for this activity, and difficulties related to obtaining behavioral health consultation and treatment from specialists. Child and adolescent psychiatrists may assist pediatric primary care practices with engaging youth and families around screening by assisting with identifying rating scales that have good psychometric characteristics across multiple languages and are validated in diverse samples and available within the public domain. Additionally, they may partner with pediatric primary care professionals to assist with optimizing screening workflows and linkage to specialized services.

Debbie H. Lu, Julie A. Dopheide, Dri Wang, Jessica K. Jeffrey, and Steven Chen

Access to mental health care is a long-standing challenge. The high, rising prevalence of mental health disorders and a shortage of mental health professionals has further strained an already fragile system. The clinical pharmacy is underutilized within the mental health space. Interdisciplinary collaboration between child psychiatrists and mental health pharmacists gives the psychiatrist more time for patient evaluation and treatment, while the psychiatric pharmacist provides drug monitoring, medication coordination, and education for providers. This collaborative approach improves outcomes, prevents adverse drug events, reduces hospital stays, lessens emergency department visits, and improves engagement and adherence.

Mark S. Borer and Susan H. McDaniel

Psychiatry and psychology have a long history of competition that too often interferes with the collaboration that can characterize complementary contributions to our common missions. We hope this article will inspire our disciplines to expand on this collaboration, for the sake of our children and families, our communities, our colleagues, and honestly, ourselves. We are better together than apart. This text is a blueprint for the assumptions, attitudes, skills, and advocacy that can make this partnership healthy and successful.

Suzie C. Nelson, Jessica K. Jeffrey, Andrew Lustbader, Jessica Rak, Mona Gandhi, Rajeev Krishna, Marcus Merriman, Vonda Keels-Lowe, and Amy Hoisington-Stabile

The unmet behavioral health treatment needs of children and adolescents have become a public health crisis in the United States, with only 20% of youths obtaining assessment and intervention when indicated. Workforce shortages, including mental health professionals who can provide pharmacologic intervention within an appropriate biopsychosocial context, directly impede our ability to address this crisis. The authors examine the history, education, regulation, and practice of psychiatric mental health nurse practitioners and consider models of practice that can be beneficial across treatment settings in order to provide better care of vulnerable youth in ways that foster partnership rather than competition.

CHILD AND ADOLESCENT PSYCHIATRIC CLINICS

SERIES OF RELATED INTEREST

Psychiatric Clinics of North America
https://www.psych.theclinics.com/
Pediatric Clinics of North America
https://www.pediatric.theclinics.com/
Neurologic Clinics
https://www.neurologic.theclinics.com/

AACAP Members: Please go to www.jaacap.org for information on access to the Child and Adolescent Psychiatric Clinics. *Resident* Members of AACAP: Special access information is available at www.childpsych.theclinics.com.

THE CLINICS ARE AVAILABLE ONLINE!
Access your subscription at:
www.theclinics.com

Preface

At the Cliff: Partnership and Collaboration to Address our Public Mental Health Crisis

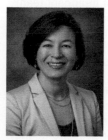 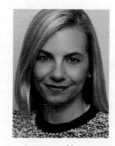 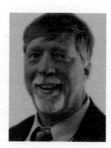 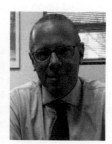

Suzie C. Nelson, MD   Jessica K. Jeffrey, MD, MPH, MBA   Mark S. Borer, MD   Barry D. Sarvet, MD

Editors

Medicine has historically called upon its professionals to respond to the evolving needs of the population and the systems in which the care of patients take place. From the time of our early development as a field of medicine in the first child guidance clinics, child and adolescent psychiatrists (CAP) have adjusted to significant change.[1,2] Movement from institutionalized to industrial settings,[3] practice under managed care,[4] and a growth of possibilities under the Affordable Care Act[5] have been a living history for CAPs who are in current practice and mentoring new practitioners today. We have been charged with being ready to face any change and advocate for our patients through it all.

We are at a precipice in medicine with an already gaping and growing mental health crisis for our nation's youth. By now, many mental health professionals are familiar with the statistics exemplifying how our current supply of every category of mental health professional is not able to meet the current demand for mental health care. Of the approximately 15 million children and adolescents in the United States who likely suffer from a behavioral health condition,[6] only 20% receive treatment.[7,8] Furthermore, that very limited care is not equitable, because racial, ethnic, and socioeconomic disparities[9] amplify the shortage of care access; among children living in poverty who need mental health services, less than 15% receive care at all and even less complete treatment.[10,11]

The recent COVID-19 global pandemic has further complicated this challenge.[12] Historical models of the impact of exposure to medical disasters are clues to the future with regard to the development of already prevalent conditions, such as depression and posttraumatic stress disorder.[13,14] Social isolation and subjective feelings of

Child Adolesc Psychiatric Clin N Am 30 (2021) xiii–xviii
https://doi.org/10.1016/j.chc.2021.07.006
1056-4993/21/© 2021 Published by Elsevier Inc.

loneliness are linked with suicidal ideation and attempt.[15] The necessity of public health measures, such as social distancing and quarantine, has contributed to long-term stress and could induce psychological sequelae that mental health professionals must be ready to address,[16,17] on top of the previously growing need for mental health services we had hoped to mitigate before a global pandemic could ever have been anticipated. Charged with the welfare of a population of children and adolescents, we attempt yet again to make rapid adjustments to meet the needs of youth and families.

Transformation of clinical practice is needed to solve the mental health crisis. CAPs are called upon in multiple clinical settings to provide leadership of treatment teams and liaise with other medical specialties to engage in patient care not only at the individual level but also at population levels. Collaborative partnerships are critical to multiply the effectiveness of each individual professional in the system of health care. Articles in this issue discuss the importance of such partnerships and provide examples of multiple collaborations and how they can transform the practice of mental health care for youth to better combat the current mental health crisis, and with time, it is hoped turn away from the crisis and move toward thriving in the care of our youth.

Our issue opens with a discussion of teamwork, a multidisciplinary view on how mental health professionals can better participate in comprehensive interagency cooperation in order to meet the common goal of improving access to quality mental health care for youth. Principles of the utility of teams, the proper formation of teams, and promotion of successful teamwork are critical foundational elements to understand as we embark on the more specific collaborations that follow. Application of successful practices in business can serve as models to help medical practice transform in ways to better serve our patients. Our own work as CAPs and other mental health professionals who specialize in helping youth provides an obvious background into the importance of a healthy developmental process; teams must also form and develop appropriately in order to be healthy and thrive in reaching shared goals. Threats toward healthy development of teams can be identified and their sequelae thwarted, similarly to our fostering healthy development in an individual. Our work in achieving positive transformation in clinical practice, namely successful collaborations toward this end, progresses more effectively when we are more familiar with the basic tenets of working in teams.

One such team model is collaborative and integrated care (CIC), and several articles examine this more closely. Is there an ethical imperative supporting increasing numbers of mental health and general medical professionals participating in these models? Ethical value models are reviewed to attempt to answer to this question. Indeed, the overall concept of collaboration (with a little "c") is one way to understand the need for working together to achieve a common goal of providing better quality mental health care for youth and families. In CIC, Collaboration (with a big "C") refers to a specific model of providing this care. Whenever multidisciplinary teams work together, there will always be guild-specific codes of ethics that each professional group is duty-bound to follow, but the authors discuss particular ethical values that are common principles among groups likely to engage in this work.

Training and education are potential launch settings for transformation of clinical practice, and the next article in this issue is a scoping review examining the literature for the use of interprofessional education (IPE) in provision of mental health care for youth. This addition to the literature, more specifically examining child mental health IPE, helps demonstrate the importance of these partnerships among various specialists from their earliest experiences in providing care. The tone for future practice and habits for establishing care are set to some degree in educational programs and postgraduate training, making these important settings for collaborative work.

In particular, for those professionals who are less familiar with child and adolescent systems of care, or perhaps as a primer for those who work more with only specific systems of care and thus have less exposure to all, the article discussing eight main child-serving systems is an important review. The perspective offered demonstrates how each system fits into overall health care delivery models in our communities. Familiarity with these systems is critical to help all mental health professionals see how each part fits into the whole spectrum of care. This is especially true when considering population-based methods both to prevent illness and to address barriers to care and when attempting to identify stakeholders that should be part of particular teams to provide mental health intervention for youth and families. At the individual level, CAPs benefit from learning how career stage can impact their viewpoints on systems of care and how they can better participate at a population health level.

Following those initial articles offering broader views for mental health professionals on how we can understand our own roles in this overarching concept of collaboration, we begin to examine specific partnerships or models of collaboration that can serve as potential blueprints for application. One such critical concept that cannot be forgotten in work with youth is the role of trauma and resilience informed care. Prevention of and interventions to address early childhood adversity are among the most critical priorities valued by child and adolescent mental health professionals. This addresses our public mental health crisis at a population level, not only by working with those who present in our traditional clinical settings with the sequelae of trauma but also by emphasizing the promotion of good mental health and being ready to address every level in between in a tiered approach. Disparities in care provision, barriers to care, and addressing social determinants of health are also important for care provision at the community or population level. That the article also provides a specific model of collaboration between a public academic university and a community mental health system is demonstrative of the type of partnership that can mutually serve both training needs and critical mental health access needs.

That the field of CAP and the dawn of school-based health services arose in a similar time in the United States is no accident, and thus, collaboration with schools is another critical population-based partnership. It is true that "school is where the children are," and thus, this setting is an ideal one in which to launch prevention, screening, and early intervention. The authors provide a historical overview of school-based health and provide the reader with key understanding of this specific system of care. That there is a strong evidence base for the positive outcomes in youth who are served by school-based health centers (SBHCs) speaks to the importance of addressing barriers to provision of care in these settings. CAPs can have a very unique type of consultation-liaison role in SBHCs as we work with our education colleagues.

Moving toward some specific medically based partnerships, the next article examines the CIC model, specifically, from the perspective of the partnership that exists between the CAP and the pediatric primary care clinician (PPCC). A growing body of literature supports increasing use of CIC, yet these models continue to face challenges with implementation and sustainability. The author provides a theoretical overview but also very practical tips for CAPs in a CIC model. Engagement in and fostering the collaborative relationship between the CAP and the PPCC are critical to the success of CIC, and by extension, meeting the goal of increasing access to mental health care for youth and families.

As a corollary to the engagement between CAPs and PPCCs, appropriate screening for behavioral health conditions using validated, using validated, with a preference for freely available, rating scales is one specific mechanism by which CAPs can support our pediatric colleagues. While universal screening is highly recommended, it is not yet consistently practiced and applied, creating a potential gap in the identification of youth in need of mental health services. A table summarizing available caregiver and youth scales and a detailed case presentation serve as tools that can foster the practice of behavioral health screening in most settings.

Another specific partnership that is growing in availability and has an established evidence base is that between psychiatrists and mental health pharmacists. This particular interdisciplinary collaboration can assist in making care more efficient, effective, and equitable. Assistance in monitoring for adverse effects and provision of medication-specific psychoeducation improve the quality of care and promise to improve treatment adherence. The authors present a comprehensive medication management model and multiple case-based demonstrations of this model for readers who look to implement it into their practice settings.

Historically, collaborations among mental health professionals have centered on relationships among the specific mental health disciplines themselves. An article specifically discussing the working relationships between psychiatrists and psychologists meets the need to more effectively collaborate head-on, by directly challenging any assertion that there should be competition between these two professions. Instead, the authors offer their blueprint for what is needed to build more effective partnerships to meet the needs of our youth and families. They summarize the varied education and training pathways between these specialties and discuss background, process, and outcomes of interprofessional teamwork within these partnerships in the context of CIC. Fostering IPE and specific efforts between national professional organizations that represent both psychiatrists and psychologists, the authors highlight the need to come together for beneficial quality mental health care of youth and families.

The issue concludes with the discussion of another specific partnership between psychiatrists and advanced practice psychiatric nurses (APPNs). Ultimately, we face a workforce shortage to meet current and future mental health needs. Several articles in this issue also quote known statistics about the shortage of psychiatrists, and particularly CAPs, to address mental health conditions in youth. A review of APPN training pathways is provided for readers less familiar with these programs. State-by-state regulatory differences and the evolution of practice regulation are also discussed in the context of impact on access to mental health intervention. The authors provide narrative descriptions of care models in varied practice settings that represent differing regions and therefore differing regulations on nurse practitioner practice. Characteristics of successful partnerships are reviewed as a means to increase access to critical mental health shortages in ways that encourage quality care and the support of CAPs partnering with APPNs. As practice evolves and regulations shift, embracing effective collegial relationships between these two professional groups can achieve their common goal to provide better care for youth and families.

In a review of mechanisms to improve access to mental health care for low-income youth and families via primary care, Hodgkinson and colleagues[18] provide a helpful summary of challenges to date, including how prior models of care have failed to prevent barriers, despite best efforts and intentions. They conclude with specific recommendations for the practice of integrating mental health services into primary care. At the level of the individual professional, interventions can be made in the arenas of "education and training, clinical infrastructure, and multidisciplinary teams." They then follow that broad recommendation with a targeted outline of more specific steps to achieve the goal of improving access to care. Their principles, however, are useful across all of the systems of care that have been discussed in this issue and among teams of professionals who are charged with improving the mental health of our youth. Ultimately, we all hold some level of individual professional responsibility to address the public mental health crisis, but the history of relying on our own individual abilities within smaller or siloed areas of responsibility has not been enough. We cannot simply work harder at that same model and expect a different result, and the collaborative partnerships discussed here are among those that have provided some promise to catch what we have heretofore missed. This need, to improve access to mental health care, is more critical than ever. We are at the cliff, and we can work together to catch, to pull back, and to turn.

Suzie C. Nelson, MD
Wright State University
Boonshoft School of Medicine
Department of Psychiatry
2555 University Boulevard
Dayton, OH 45324, USA

Jessica K. Jeffrey, MD, MPH, MBA
Department of Psychiatry and Biobehavioral Sciences
University of California, Los Angeles
760 Westwood Plaza, Room A7-372
Los Angeles, CA 90095, USA

Mark S. Borer, MD
Psychiatric Access for Central Delaware, P.A.
Board Certified Child and Adolescent
General Adult Psychiatry; Family Psychiatry
846 Walker Road, Ste 32-2
Dover, DE 19904, USA

Barry D. Sarvet, MD
Department of Psychiatry
University of Massachusetts Medical
School-Baystate
Baystate Medical Center
759 Chestnut Street, WG703
Springfield, MA 01199, USA

E-mail addresses:
suzie.nelson@wright.edu (S.C. Nelson)
jjeffrey@mednet.ucla.edu (J.K. Jeffrey)
bugglinborer@comcast.net (M.S. Borer)
barry.sarvet@baystatehealth.org (B.D. Sarvet)

REFERENCES

1. Mian AI, Milavic G, Skokauskas N. Child and adolescent psychiatry training: a global perspective. Child Adolesc Psychiatr Clin N Am 2015;24(4):699–714.

2. Beuttler F, Bell C. For the welfare of every child—a brief history of the Institute for Juvenile Research, 1909–2010. Chicago: University of Illinois; 2010.

3. Bittker TE. The industrialization of American psychiatry. Am J Psychiatry 1985; 142(2):149–54.

4. Rosenberg E, DeMaso DR. A doubtful guest: managed care and mental health. Child Adolesc Psychiatr Clin N Am 2008;17(1):53–66.

5. Rozensky RH. Implications of the Patient Protection and Affordable Care Act: preparing the professional psychology workforce for primary care. Prof Psychol Res Pr 2014;45:200–11. https://doi.org/10.1037/a0036550.

6. Perou R, Bitsko RH, Blumberg SJ, et al. Mental health surveillance among children—United States, 2005–2011. MMWR Suppl 2013;62(2):1–35.

7. US Department of Health Human Services. Mental health: a report of the surgeon general. Rockville, MD: US Department of Health and Human Services, Substance Abuse and Mental Health Services Administration, Center for Mental Health Services, National Institutes of Health, National Institute of Mental Health; 1999.

8. Whitney D, Peterson M. US national and state-level prevalence of mental health disorders and disparities of mental health care use in children. JAMA Pediatr 2019;173(4):389–91. https://doi.org/10.1001/jamapediatrics.2018.5399.

9. Alegria M, Vallas M, Pumariega AJ. Racial and ethnic disparities in pediatric mental health. Child Adolesc Psychiatr Clin N Am 2010;19(4):759–74.

10. Kataoka SH, Zhang L, Wells KB. Unmet need for mental health care among US children: variation by ethnicity and insurance status. Am J Psychiatry 2002; 159(9):1548–55.

11. Santiago CD, Kaltman S, Miranda J. Poverty and mental health: how do low-income adults and children fare in psychotherapy? J Clin Psychol 2013;69(2): 115–26.

12. Marques de Miranda D, da Silva Athanasio B, Sena Oliveira AC, et al. How is COVID-19 pandemic impacting mental health of children and adolescents? Int J Disaster Risk Reduct 2020;51:101845. https://doi.org/10.1016/j.ijdrr.2020. 101845. Epub 2020 Sep 10. PMID: 32929399; PMCID: PMC7481176.

13. Liu X, Kakade M, Fuller CJ, et al. Depression after exposure to stressful events: lessons learned from the severe acute respiratory syndrome epidemic. Compr Psychiatry 2012;53(1):15–23.

14. Sprang G, Silman M. Posttraumatic stress disorder in parents and youth after health-related disasters. Disaster Med Public Health Prep 2013;7(1):105–10.

15. Calati R, Ferrari C, Brittner M, et al. Suicidal thoughts and behaviors and social isolation: a narrative review of the literature. J Affect Disord 2019;245:653–67.

16. Brooks SK, Webster RK, Smith LE, et al. The psychological impact of quarantine and how to reduce it: rapid review of the evidence. Lancet 2020;395(10227): 912–20.

17. Wang G, Zhang Y, Zhao J, et al. Mitigate the effects of home confinement on children during the COVID-19 outbreak. Lancet 2020;395(10228):945–7.

18. Hodgkinson S, Godoy L, Beers LS, et al. Improving mental health access for low-income children and families in the primary care setting. Pediatrics 2017;139(1): e20151175.

Teamwork
A Multidisciplinary Review

William Clark, MD, MBA

KEYWORDS

- Teams • Teamwork • Collaboration • Team development • Integrated care
- Mental health

KEY POINTS

- Teamwork is needed to bridge growing gaps in access to mental health care.
- When properly used, teams can be effective at solving unique and complex problems.
- A team requires clearly defined members with diverse perspectives and skills.
- Understanding the different stages or dimensions of a team can help to guide team-based interventions and move toward a more productive form of teamwork.
- Effective teamwork requires fostering a collaborative environment. Organizations should embrace a culture of continuous improvement to adapt to change.

INTRODUCTION

Creative solutions are needed to address growing gaps in mental health care.[1] Disparities in accessing quality mental health care have only become more apparent in the context of a global pandemic.[2] Already stretched resources have been further stressed, with increasing demand to provide child and adolescent patients with proper mental health care.[3,4] The pandemic has simultaneously decreased access to mental health services, as well as increased demand for appropriate mental health care.[5] There is an increasing need for expanding access to care through the use of collaborative mental health care models. Interdisciplinary teamwork through collaborative care models has arguably become an emerging best practice in mental health care.[6,7] And, according to the American Academy of Child and Adolescent Psychiatry, the evolving standard of care requires multidisciplinary collaboration with a mandate for comprehensive interagency cooperation.[8]

This article summarizes the existing multidisciplinary literature on teamwork, primarily from a business and health care perspective. Although this review is targeted toward health care professionals, the principles are widely applicable across disciplines. I invite you to consider this review when framing current and future team efforts. As leaders of collaborative teams, once we understand the boundaries

Department of Psychiatry, Wright State University, Wright-Patterson Medical Center, Mental Health Clinic, 4th Floor, 4881 Sugar Maple Avenue, WPAFB, OH 45433, USA
E-mail addresses: William.r.clark@wright.edu; William.r.clark305.mil@mail.mil

Child Adolesc Psychiatric Clin N Am 30 (2021) 685–695
https://doi.org/10.1016/j.chc.2021.05.003
1056-4993/21/Published by Elsevier Inc.
childpsych.theclinics.com

and mechanisms of an effective team, we can develop a framework that fosters collaboration and optimizes team effectiveness. We will then review evidence-based techniques and expert opinions for building and managing successful teams that can be applied to a variety of health care-related settings.

WHAT MAKES A TEAM?

It is important to first carefully define and evaluate whether a team is the right mechanism for accomplishing a task or goal. Colloquially, a team is simply a group of people working together. However, this definition is insufficient for helping to guide the development of an effective team.[9] Experts in studying teamwork and team development tend to emphasize several key components that help differentiate teams from other forms of working groups, parallel groups, partnerships, and so on.

First, teamwork involves a group with commitment to a shared purpose or goal. This goal can differ from typical working groups that involve a shared project; however, each individual in a working group is accountable only to themselves and their contribution. Individuals in a working group may only be motivated to accomplish their personal task without concern for the overall mission of the project.[9,10] In a team, it is important for all members to develop a shared purpose that drives individual and group achievement.

Effective teams have individual as well as mutual accountability for success. Owing to a shared commitment, team members not only want to succeed in their own personal performance, they also have a stake in the overall outcome of the team.[9] They may be willing to sacrifice some personal reward for the better success of the mission. This collaboration occurs because of a shared purpose.

To achieve greater success from teamwork, we need members with diverse perspectives and skills.[11] Working groups and other forms of parallel working environments may have a number of people working on similar functions with similar perspectives to accomplish joint tasks. Tasks are completed in a team through joint collaborative effort that uses diverse perspectives and skills to develop more creative and unique solutions that cannot be accomplished individually.[9,10]

Last, a team requires appropriate ground rules and boundaries. A team needs clearly defined members, preferably a small number of people, for members to mature into their respective team roles. Rules for operation are required to ensure the team functions in a safe, predictable, and manageable fashion.[9,10] Boundaries and consistency help team members to develop the trust in each other that leads to increased creativity and perceived meaningfulness.[9,10] All teams require some boundaries or rules to operate effectively.

SHOULD WE USE A TEAM?

It is important that we determine the most appropriate organizational mechanism for accomplishing our goals. We must ask ourselves if we truly need to develop a team for our goal. Given the extensive emphasis on teamwork, we may be fooled into creating unnecessary teams when other means of completing tasks may be more effective and easier to implement.[12] True teamwork can provide exceptional solutions; however, it also requires a significant amount of additional time and resources to develop. When teams are ineffectively formed, they can be worse at accomplishing tasks, even compared with a single individual.[12] We should reserve the use of teams for situations that require creative and novel solutions to complex problems that would likely not be possible through individual means.[13] We are expecting teams, through collaborative efforts, to produce more than the sum of its parts.

If the task at hand requires a complex and creative solution, next we need to determine if we have the resources to support a team effort. An effective team will require a small group of individuals with complementary skills, likely from a variety of disciplines. It can be challenging to provide the necessary resources to support interdisciplinary collaboration. Teams require significant amounts of time to interact, develop, and mature to work collaboratively.[14] This time can be costly when it takes away focus and energy from other responsibilities.[9] This process can create friction between competing team assignments and result in other opportunity costs.[9] A team also requires physical or virtual space to interact. This space can be difficult to provide for team members who may not have consistent availability or might be distributed far from one another geographically.[15] Some form of synchronous communication is likely required for effective teamwork. There are a number of practical considerations needed before committing to the development of a truly collaborative effort.

We should also determine if our individual team members will be able to commit the time needed to see the development of team collaboration. If we will not be able to maintain consistent involvement, the group dynamic will struggle to form adequate social boundaries and expectations that aid in collaborative activities.[14] Without consistent involvement of the same participants, the group will not have a chance to develop into a fully collaborative team.

Most important, we need to find team members with a common set of values and purpose to drive accountability and motivation. There needs to be a balance between team members that share similar values while simultaneously sharing different perspectives. This point should underscore the importance of developing a diverse workforce or organization for which teamwork can be used more effectively.[11,16] If we do not have consistent members with diverse perspectives to pool from, we likely cannot develop a particularly fruitful team.

HOW TO BUILD A TEAM
Find the Right People

The process of developing a team capable of exceptional ingenuity can be hard to fully define from start to finish. A frequent misstep in team development is to start with goals and vision before even assembling the key members of the group. Some researchers of corporate success suggest that the most crucial element of team development is identifying the right people.[17] Starting with talented individuals, we can rely on team members to collaboratively develop unified goals. In situations where the problem and solution are clearly defined, a more structured group dynamic is preferred, such as a working group with clearly delegated roles. A team structure is best for identifying solutions to complex and unique problems. For teams to be truly collaborative, with individual and group accountability, there needs to be shared responsibility for the development of team goals and vision. We need to find the right people with a diverse and complementary set of skills and perspectives that will likely help to identify and solve complex problems.[11,16] In addition to talented and trustworthy team members, it is important to actively involve appropriate stakeholders.[18] Without the best people for the job, we are unlikely to achieve exceptional results.

Create a Framework

Once we have the right team members, it is important to provide the structure, framework, and resources required for the team to operate effectively. We start with addressing practical matters, such as determining the real or virtual space in which we will work. A clearly defined space can be virtual meeting room platforms, physical offices, or any agreed upon space in which members feel comfortable to collaborate.[19] There should be clearly defined rules of conduct. Some of these rules can be outlined for the group ahead of time, whereas other customs and courtesies should be discussed and agreed upon by team members. Giving the group a framework provides a sense of familiarity, predictability, and safety to explore tasks in creative ways without fear of judgment.[12,19,20] It is important to establish rules and expectations for communication outside of meetings between team members. And, ultimately, a leadership structure should be clearly defined.[18]

Define a Collaborative Vision and Mission

Now that we have identified the members of our team and basic ground rules, we can start to develop a detailed vision and mission. There is evidence that individuals remain more motivated when they are involved in the collaborative development of the group mission.[21,22] The terms "vision" and "mission" are often used interchangeably; however, it can be helpful to be more intentional with these terms to help further develop more detailed and actionable goals. The vision is the long-term ideal outcome of the organization.[18] The vision is a stretch of what the organization aspires to become and achieve. The mission of an organization is the main goal that has been identified and will subsequently be broken down into actionable tasks that can be measured, evaluated, and achieved.[18] If we have assembled the right team members, they should be in the position to make the best decisions on the team's vision, mission, and goals. A good team manager supports the group's direction, but he or she also ensures the team is identifying specific, measurable, achievable, relevant, and timely (SMART) goals.[18] It is important to take time as a team to collaboratively develop the mission and goals so that we can keep the group moving toward success.

HOW DOES TEAMWORK DEVELOP?

Conceptualizing team development allows team members and leaders to better understand the state of the team and how it can expect to mature. Understanding the steps that teams take throughout development helps to prepare and predict foreseeable complications that may hinder the success of projects and goals. Understanding the progression of development also helps us to understand where we are in that process so that we can better understand how our team compares with other successful groups. A team may, for example, be struggling to understand power dynamics as well as implicit and explicit roles. Acknowledging that this may be a normal part of team development may help to maintain morale among the group and keep members future oriented. There are a number of theories that attempt to explain the maturation of teams with similar stages or dimensions. Most theorists agree with the importance of a mutually developed team culture among members to reach higher levels of performance. However, there is some debate about the linearity of progression through stages versus character dimensions that may best describe how teams operate over time.

Tuckman's Team Development Model

The most widely cited team theory is Tuckman's model, which describes group development in fairly linear developmental stages. Tuckman's model synthesized a number of studies looking at group development and identified 5 common stages that were summarized as: forming, storming, norming, performing, and adjourning.[23,24] During the first stage, forming, team members may be apprehensive to assert themselves until they have a better understanding of what to expect from others in the group as well as the teams objectives. Leaders should assist the team in getting to know each other and developing a collaborative mission. During the storming stage, there is often inter-group conflict as members are starting to assert themselves, causing tensions to rise. Team members may feel frustrated with the increase in conflict. Therefore, promoting communication and diverse perspectives between team members is important during this stage. The norming stage introduces a time when team members are becoming more comfortable with each other owing to a better understanding of interpersonal re-lationships and team roles. Members become more invested in the group's mission. Now team members are able to express themselves more easily and team members are able to exchange ideas more freely, which leads to increased collaboration, in the performing stage. Revised models have included the fifth stage of adjourning, which describes the characteristics of a group's conclusion.[24] Although this is not a causal theory of group development, it does have useful descriptions of what to expect as teams evolve.

Informal Role Theory

An alternative description of team development, called informal role theory, concep-tualizes the group structure as a set of interdependent informal roles.[25] It defines an informal role as a pattern of interpersonal behavior that a team comes to expect from a team member. The theory proposes that team development can be understood through analyzing the patterns of these informal roles at different time points.[25] During the forming stages of team development, this theory describes individual team mem-bers as largely isolated owing to team ambiguity and confusion. This process can result in conflict over areas of authority and control. A combination of factors, including inherent personalities, stereotyping, and projection, contribute to members interacting in recognizable patterns early in team development. The authors of this theory pro-pose a few typical informal roles: superhero, tyrant, leader's helper, peacemaker, lightning rod, and scapegoat.[25] The superhero and tyrant are both seen as dominant characters. However, the superhero is viewed as competent, dedicated, and hard working, whereas the tyrant is seen as oppressive and hostile by other team members. Depending on how a team member may typically address conflict-related anxiety, they may take on a particularly helpful role or routinely pacify the situation. A team member may unconsciously seek to mitigate group tension by acting as a lightning rod by challenging authority and drawing conflict away from others. Often during con-flict and uncertainty, a less competent team member may become the scapegoat of the group as a means of displacing anger and responsibility. Ultimately, the informal role theory argues that, as the team evolves, these informal roles become less distinct and interpersonal behavior becomes more uniform.[25] As ambiguity among the team decreases, so do general anxiety and ego defenses. Team members become more group oriented and adopt a shared team culture. As a result of this advanced stage, team members are able to operate more collaboratively and productively.

Team Empowerment Theory

A less linear theory of team development conceptualizes stages in terms of empow-erment. These stages may be better conceptualized as team dimensions that are continuously changing over time. This theory defines 4 stages: job enlargement, job enrichment, cooperation, and high performance.[26] In a state of job enlargement, the team is focused on acquiring technical and conceptual knowledge of all the roles within the team. During job enrichment, the team is taking on more autonomous man-agement of tasks. The team becomes more self-reliant as a result of improved communication and collaboration during the stage of cooperation. Finally, the team has reached a stage of high performance when it is capable of solving nonroutine problems and the group is focused on organizational performance over individual achievement. Research on the empowerment theory suggested a nonlinear pattern of development among various types of teams.[26] It seems that promoting the dimensions of job enlargement and job enrichment improve team member satisfaction.[26] Research also underscores the necessity of cooperation for reaching higher levels of achievement. The empowerment theory for describing team dimensions can help leaders to identify ways to improve team satisfaction and productivity by promoting strategies that train and involve the entire team.

Despite several theories describing team development, many of the stages and dimensions that have been observed overlap conceptually. For groups to develop into highly successful teams, there seems to be a progression beginning with developing an understanding of team roles and its mission. Fostering communication seems to be critical for reaching higher levels of team performance, which may entail periods of increased tension within the group. When teams are in a high performing stage, all members share a mutual respect and understanding that enhances communication and productive exchange of diverse perspectives.

HOW TO PROMOTE SUCCESSFUL TEAMWORK
Establish Leadership

Leadership should be structured based on the needs of each unique team. Even the most autonomous teams benefit from some formal established leadership. The leader's role is not to determine the goals or how to achieve them. However, a leader is responsible for ensuring a team stays resourced and motivated. Leaders helps the organization to navigate through the various stages of team development. An effective team leader ensures that all the right people are involved, all the needs of the team are met, and that the team continues to work toward self-determined goals.[18] An expert in collaboration research contends that effective leaders are authentically interested in diverse insights, willing to explore conflicting opinions, and heavily invested in group success.[27] Some companies have gone so far as to structure a culture of corporate liberation, in which teams have the freedom to take action for the best interest of the organization. These companies manage operations by encouraging employee-driven solutions with resource support provided by leadership.[22] And in line with this philosophy, "Good to Great" leaders make decisive actions about who joins the team, but they provide the freedom for the team members to decide how to accomplish the mission.[17] Even with a highly autonomous team, it is helpful to identify formal leadership to ensure the team stays on task, motivated, and adequately resourced.

Support a Collaborative Environment

One of the most important factors for successful collaboration is effective communication. for team members to share ideas and develop innovative solutions, there needs to be effective open communication. One study found a strong positive association between the level of energy and engagement involved in team communication patterns and organizational success.[28,29] The mode of communication also impacts team success. Research, before the global pandemic, emphasized the importance of face-to-face interactions as opposed to email and electronic messaging.[29] Even though email can help to maintain connections within the group, it seems to have limitations for promoting truly creative and collaborative environments. Subsequent studies need to be conducted to determine the ability of video conferences to foster collaboration as compared with in-person working environments.

Effective communication between team members requires trust rooted in individual and group emotional intelligence. Individual emotional intelligence is the ability to relate to others and exhibit consistent affective self-regulation. Some experts believe emotional intelligence is as important as the intelligence quotient in predicting individual effectiveness.[19] Groups also exhibit forms of emotional intelligence that are more than the sum of its members. Group emotional intelligence has been shown to be an important factor in promoting collaboration.[30] It can be promoted through team norms that support an awareness and regulation of emotions within and outside the team. This factor means allowing emotions within the team to be identified and addressed in a nonjudgmental and nonthreatening manner.[19,30] Practicing empathy within the group enhances trust and communication, leading to a higher functioning team.

Closely related to emotional intelligence, social intelligence is another set of skills that can be cultivated to promote enhanced communication within teams. Social intelligence is more relationship based and uses neurobiology to help explain the ability for 1 individual to influence the feelings of another.[31] Emotional intelligence allows one to identify and regulate emotions, whereas social intelligence is an understanding of social dynamics. When focused, these skills can be used to more effectively connect and communicate with the rest of the team. Social intelligence also assists in the vital role of managing team conflict in a healthy and productive way. Some research suggests that social intelligence is even more predictive of performance than emotional intelligence.[31]

Embracing diverse perspectives is incredibly valuable for promoting a collaborative environment. Recruiting diverse team members will be ineffective if their differing skills and perspectives are not embraced throughout the creative process. Often, conflict can be seen as disruptive; however, handled constructively, it can enhance the creative nature of teams to identify novel solutions to complex problems. It is vital to separate interpersonal conflict from professional conflict.[16] One research group suggests encouraging constructive conflict by focusing on issues instead of personalities, framing decisions as collaborations toward achieving group goals, and establishing a sense of fairness and equity in the decision-making process.[16]

It can be helpful to implement team-building interventions throughout the life of a team to promote a healthy collaborative environment. This practice may include initial trainings as well as periodic team-building exercises. These initiatives have been shown to be helpful in preparing teams for stressful emergency situations in a variety of disciplines.[32,33] There are also plenty of anecdotal reports and expert opinions about the impact of team-building interventions in more routine and collaborative settings.[18] It is likely that team building interventions can be effective for enhancing interpersonal communication, social and emotional intelligence, and dealing with conflict resolution.

Maintain Motivation

Successful teams are able to maintain individual and group motivation by staying focused on the meaningfulness of the work, breaking down goals into specific actionable steps, and structuring team-based incentives for performance.[13] Multiple studies across various disciplines support the importance of meaningfulness as a prerequisite for short and long-term motivation.[34] Meaningfulness is more easily maintained when goals are broken down into multiple, readily achievable steps, and individuals or teams are given the autonomy to decide how best to accomplish goals. It is also important for all members of the team to know how their work contributes to the overall mission.[35] Evidence also suggests that groups are more successful when motivated by team-based performance incentives.[36] For a team to maintain success over time, there need to be strategic efforts to address fluctuations in team motivation.

Promote Continuous Improvement

The success of long-term organizations relies on their ability to identify areas for improvement and embrace change. Team performance should be measured based on its unique tasks and achievement. These measures should be identified during the planning stages as the mission and specific goals are established. Lean and Six Sigma continuous improvement process analysis tools have been adopted in a variety of industries with positive impacts on performance.[18] Lean process analysis can be used for eliminating wasteful processes, whereas Six Sigma techniques are used primarily for minimizing variation within a service or product. Both of these continuous improvement processes can be established to improve quality and performance of teams in a variety of settings. There are a variety of tools used to measure how a team is functioning to better predict outcomes.[37] Team performance can also be measured within a team overtime or compared with other teams of similar structure and objectives. Continuous improvement processes should be embedded in the culture of the team to promote high standards and the expectation of an adaptable organization.[18] Continuous improvement processes, as well as team-enhancing exercises, can be used to promote a culture of flexibility and success regardless of inevitable changes.[38]

CASE EXAMPLE

The hospital administrators for a major nonprofit hospital system have been receiving consistent feedback from primary care providers that there are significant delays in meeting mental health referral demands. Primary care providers and their patients have been feeling frustrated by extended wait times to connect with a psychiatrist in the hospital system and the surrounding community. After discussions with hospital psychiatrists, the administrators confirm there are limited available appointments and not enough psychiatrists to cover current demands.

One of the current consult and liaison psychiatrists in the hospital offers her time to assist in an outpatient integrated mental health care initiative to increase access to outpatient psychiatric care. In an attempt to be proactive, an administrator takes on the role of coordinating this initiative by arranging a space and time once a week for the psychiatrist to be present in the outpatient primary care clinic attached to the main hospital. Several expected technical and administrative issues arose at the first scheduled visit to the primary care clinic; however, everyone in the clinic was already busy with their own patients and the psychiatrist did not have a good contact person for addressing these issues.

A month later, the psychiatrist finally straightened out technical issues with the electronic medical record and clinic-specific details; however, more systemic issues are becoming apparent. There is growing resentment within the clinic about the psychiatrist's role and availability. There have been passive aggressive comments between the psychiatrist and primary care provider regarding denied referrals and lack of availability. It turns out that the majority of the primary care providers are not in the clinic the same afternoon allocated for the psychiatrist, decreasing chances for interactions and communication. The psychiatrist is frustrated with referrals that she feels could be handled by the primary care providers, and primary care providers feel the psychiatrist is trying to reject these referrals. There seem to be unclear goals for the initiative and poor communication among the providers. The psychiatrist is starting to regret having volunteered to participate in this initiative and is even considering leaving her current position in the hospital.

Based on key points from this review on teamwork, there are a number of opportunities for improving the implementation of this integrated care initiative. Ideally, the initiative would have begun with a meeting of all necessary stakeholders to agree on a primary mission. If all partners involved are in agreement with the mission, then subsequent decisions are likely to be more collaborative. Including input from all stakeholders helps to prevent some of the miscommunications and poor scheduling that occurred in this case. Increasing communication between the psychiatrist and primary care providers is likely to have a dramatic impact on program effectiveness. In this specific case, perhaps the clinic schedule could still be changed or a weekly meeting time could be established for promoting communication between providers. Not only is it possible to expand access to psychiatry with clinic time, but if aligned with the collaborative program mission, perhaps the psychiatrist could also share additional teaching points on treating psychiatric conditions. By improving primary care provider knowledge and confidence through collaboration and communication in the clinic, access to mental health care can be extended to more patients. Undoubtedly, there are many unique solutions to improving similar programs when approached from a truly collaborative perspective.

SUMMARY

Effective teamwork can help to solve unique complex problems. At times, truly collaborative work can seem difficult to reach and even harder to maintain, but applying some basic tips from team development research can help to optimize teamwork. Collaborative team efforts are especially critical for addressing the complex gaps in national and global mental health.[7,39] Because of diverse perspectives and experiences various mental health providers bring to a collaborative treatment team, there is large creative potential If we work together. Integrated mental health practices should use, and continue to research, best practices to enhance collaboration and effectiveness.

DISCLOSURE

The views expressed in this review do not reflect official policy or position of the United States Air Force. There are no personal or financial conflicts to disclose.

REFERENCES

1. Data and Statistics on Children's mental health | CDC. Centers for Disease control and prevention. 2021. Available at: https://www.cdc.gov/childrensmentalhealth/data.html. Accessed March 5, 2021.
2. Choi K, Heilemann M, Fauer A, et al. A second pandemic: mental health spillover from the novel coronavirus (COVID-19). J Am Psychiatr Nurses Assoc 2020;26(4): 340–3.
3. Henderson MD. The COVID-19 pandemic and the impact on child mental health: a socio-ecological perspective. Pediatr Nurs 2020;46(6):267–90. Accessed March 5, 2021.
4. Waselewski EA, Waselewski ME, Chang T. Needs and coping behaviors of youth in the U.S. during COVID-19. J Adolesc Health 2020;67(5):649–52.
5. Moreno C, Wykes T, Galderisi S, et al. How mental health care should change as a consequence of the COVID-19 pandemic. Lancet Psychiatry 2020;7(9):813–24.
6. Greidanus E, Warren C, Harris GE, et al. Collaborative practice in counselling: a scoping review. J Interprof Care 2020;34(3):353–61.
7. Kossaify A, Hleihel W, Lahoud J-C. Team-based efforts to improve quality of care, the fundamental role of ethics, and the responsibility of health managers:

monitoring and management strategies to enhance teamwork. Public Health 2017;153:91–8.

8. Training Toolkit for Systems-based practice. 2021. Available at: Aacap.org; https://www.aacap.org/AACAP/Resources_for_Primary_Care/Training_Toolkit_for_Systems_Based_Practice.aspx. Accessed March 5, 2021.

9. Katzenbach JR, Smith DK. The discipline of teams. Harv Bus Rev 1993;71(2):111–20.

10. Katzenbach JR, Smith DK. The discipline of Teams: a mindbook-workbook for delivering small group performance. Wiley; 2001.

11. Horwitz SK, Horwitz IB. The effects of team diversity on team outcomes: a meta-analytic review of team demography. J Management 2007;33(6):987–1015.

12. Hackman JR. Leading teams: setting the stage for great performances. Harvard Business School Press; 2002.

13. Amabile TM, Kramer SJ. The power of small wins. Harv Bus Rev 2011;89(5):70–80.

14. Pomare C, Long JC, Ellis LA, et al. Interprofessional collaboration in mental health settings: a social network analysis. J Interprof Care 2019;33(5):497–503.

15. Margolis K, Kelsay K, Talmi A, et al. A multidisciplinary, team-based teleconsultation approach to enhance child mental health services in rural pediatrics. J Educ Psychol Consultation 2018;28(3):342–67.

16. Eisenhardt KM, Kahwajy JL, Bourgeois LJ III. How management teams can have a good fight. Harv Bus Rev 1997;75(4):77–85.

17. Collins JC. Good to great: why some companies make the leap–and others don't. 1st edition. HarperBusiness; 2001.

18. White KR, Griffith JR. The well-managed healthcare organization. 8th edition. Health Administration Press; 2016.

19. Druskat VU, Wolff SB, Messer TE, et al. Team emotional intelligence: linking team social and emotional environment to team effectiveness. DIEM: Dubrovnik International Economic Meeting. January 2017:433–54.

20. Quick KS, Feldman MS. Boundaries as junctures: collaborative boundary work for building efficient resilience. J Public Adm Res Theor 2014;24(3):673–95.

21. Adler P, Hecksher C, Prusak L. Building a collaborative enterprise. Harv Bus Rev 2011;89(7/8):94–101.

22. Carney B, Getz I. Give your team the freedom to do the work they think matters most. Harvard Business Review Digital Articles. 2018:5–7.

23. Tuckman BW. Developmental sequence in small groups. Psychol Bull 1965;63:384–99.

24. Tuckman BW, Jensen MAC. Stages of small-group development revisited. Group Facilitation: A Research & Applications Journal 2010;10:43–8.

25. Farrell MP, Schmitt MH, Heinemann GD. Informal roles and the stages of interdisciplinary team development. J Interprof Care 2001;15(3):281–95.

26. Kuipers BS, de Witte MC. Teamwork: a case study on development and performance. Int J Hum Resource Manag 2005;16(2):185–201.

27. Abele J. Bringing minds together. Harv Bus Rev 2011;89(7/8):86–93.

28. Lederman O, Calacci D, MacMullen A, et al. "Sandy." Open badges: a low-cost toolkit for measuring team communication and dynamics. 2017.

29. Sandy PA. The new science of building great teams. Harv Bus Rev 2012;90(4):60–70.

30. Lin CP, He H, Baruch Y, et al. The effect of team affective tone on team performance: the roles of team identification and team cooperation. Hum Resource Manag 2017;56(6):931–52.

31. Goleman D. Social intelligence : the new science of human relationships. Bantam Books; 2006.
32. Shuffler M, Diazgranados D, Maynard M, et al. Developing, sustaining, and maximizing team effectiveness: an integrative, dynamic perspective of team development interventions. Acad Manag Ann 2018;12(2):688–724.
33. Varpio L, Bader KS, Meyer HS, et al. Interprofessional healthcare teams in the military: a scoping literature review. Mil Med 2018;183(11–12):e448–54.
34. Terry V, Sandoval A, Garza J, et al. What drives members of an interprofessional care team: a sense of self. J Interprof Educ Pract 2018;13:27–32.
35. Gulati R. Silo busting. Harv Bus Rev 2007;85(5):98–108.
36. Garbers Y, Konradt U. The effect of financial incentives on performance: a quantitative review of individual and team-based financial incentives. J Occup Organizational Psychol 2014;87(1):102–37.
37. Rousseau C, Laurin-Lamothe A, Nadeau L, et al. Measuring the quality of interprofessional collaboration in child mental health collaborative care. Int J Integrated Care 2012;12:1–8.
38. Randall JJ, Head A. Taking conversations forward: a systemic exercise for teams threatened by service restructures. J Fam Ther 2018;40(3):447–58.
39. Butler DJ, Fons D, Fisher T, et al. A review of the benefits and limitations of a primary care-embedded psychiatric consultation service in a medically underserved setting. Int J Psychiatry Med 2018;53(5/6):415–26.

Ethical Imperatives for Participation in Integrated/ Collaborative Care Models for Pediatric Mental Health Care

Shannon L. Mazur, DO, MA[a],*, Gail A. Edelsohn, MD, MSPH[b],
Peter A. DePergola II, PhD, MTS[c,d,e], Barry D. Sarvet, MD, DFAPA[f]

KEYWORDS

- Collaborative care • Integrated care • Ethics • Mental health • Pediatric
- Behavioral health

KEY POINTS

- A widespread shortage of child and adolescent psychiatrists has led to the development of clinical models for incorporating mental health treatment into primary care.
- A careful ethical analysis of integrated/collaborative care models is essential to protect the social and emotional health and safety of children with mental illness.
- Utilitarianism, political liberalism, and the theory of proportionate reason support the use of integrated/collaborative care models.
- A deontological perspective does not endorse the use of integrated/collaborative care models per se; however, moral duties derived from deontology can provide ethical guidance to the team.

INTRODUCTION

Most of the children and adolescents in the United States with serious mental health conditions do not receive timely mental health treatment.[1] One of the most significant barriers to accessing mental health care is the well-documented shortage of child and adolescent psychiatrists.[2] Other factors include persistent stigma surrounding mental

[a] Department of Psychological Medicine, Yale New Haven Hospital, 20 York Street, Fitkin 607, New Haven, CT 06510, USA; [b] Community Care Behavioral Health Organization, UPMC Insurance Services Division, 1 East Uwchlan Avenue, Suite 311, Exton, PA 19341, USA; [c] Department of Medicine, University of Massachusetts Medical School – Baystate, 759 Chestnut Street, Daly 6100B, Springfield, MA 01199, USA; [d] Department of Bioethics and Medical Humanities, College of Our Lady of the Elms, 291 Springfield Street, Chicopee, MA 01013, USA; [e] St. Augustine Center for Ethics, Religion, and Culture, College of Our Lady of the Elms, 291 Springfield Street, Chicopee, MA 01013, USA; [f] Department of Psychiatry, University of Massachusetts Medical School – Baystate, 759 Chestnut Street, WG703, Springfield, MA 01199, USA
* Corresponding author.
E-mail address: Shannon.Mazur@yale.edu

Child Adolesc Psychiatric Clin N Am 30 (2021) 697–712
https://doi.org/10.1016/j.chc.2021.06.001
1056-4993/21/© 2021 Elsevier Inc. All rights reserved.

illness, inadequate funding of mental health services, lack of screening, and limited public awareness and education about mental illness. In response to this problem, clinical models for incorporating mental health treatment into pediatric primary care services, designed for improving access to care for children, have been rapidly proliferating. Integrating mental health into primary care is attractive for several reasons[3]: (1) primary care serves as the hub of the health care system with the essential responsibility of screening, health promotion, and coordination of care; (2) primary care providers are much more accessible than specialists and highly trusted by parents; (3) incorporating mental health into primary care emphasizes the interdependence of mental and physical health and has been found to improve physical health outcomes; and (4) addressing mental health concerns in the primary care setting has a normalizing impact and thereby may reduce stigma. The growth of integrated and collaborative practices of mental health care delivery in primary care has been associated with an increase in value-based payment models as well as increasing societal recognition of the importance of mental health to general health.

Different approaches for the integration of mental health care into primary care have been proposed; however, 3 models have become most prevalent. Models vary according to resources within the practice, external resources available to the practice, and methods of incorporating the involvement of specialists (**Table 1**). In the *Behavioral Health Consultant* (BHC) model, also referred to as the Primary Care Behavioral Health model, health care practices have an embedded licensed behavioral health clinician, usually a clinical social worker or psychologist, continually available to address mental health presentations in the practice, providing consultations, brief counseling, and coordinating referrals to external specialists.[4] In the *Child Psychiatry Access Program* (CPAP) model, teams of child and adolescent psychiatrists and other mental health providers establish collaborative relationships with pediatric primary care teams throughout a geographic region to provide immediate telephone consultation, expedite outpatient psychiatric evaluation, assist with referral for specialty mental health resources, and deliver continuing education.[5] The *Collaborative Care* model is an evidence-based model for providing treatment to patients with mild/moderate disorders in the primary care setting.[6] In this model, an embedded behavioral health clinician/care manager, an external consulting psychiatrist, and the primary care provider work as a team, while using standardized clinical measures to guide pediatric mental health treatment.

A recent meta-analysis demonstrated that adequately resourced, integrated behavioral health programs in the pediatric primary care setting are associated with improved clinical outcomes compared with usual care.[7] Formal assessment of the CPAP model revealed widespread utilization and associated improved confidence and engagement with pediatric primary care providers (PPCPs) delivering mental health care.[8] Parents report high levels of satisfaction in the performance of their PPCP when delivering mental health services with the support of a CPAP.[9]

An overarching principle common to all models of integrated and collaborative care is that the primary care team assumes ownership and responsibility for addressing mental health needs for patients in their panel. This role includes detection, initial assessment, development and implementation of a treatment plan, coordination of referrals to specialists as needed, and monitoring progress. In contrast, within a traditional care model the PPCP may try to address behavioral health concerns as they arise; however, these issues are not considered a core responsibility of the practice. Often, PPCPs are without an organized approach and specific resources for performing this function. In this respect, integrated or collaborative models of mental health care in primary care practice represent a shift in responsibility from the child and

Table 1 Models of behavioral health integration in pediatric primary care			
	Behavioral Health Consultant (BHC) Model	**Child Psychiatry Access Programs (CPAP)**	**Collaborative Care Model (CCM)**
Behavioral health team	On site: behavioral health clinician (social worker, psychologist, nurse practitioner)	Off-site: mental health team (child and adolescent psychiatrists, other behavioral health clinicians, care coordinator)	On site: behavioral health clinician/care manager Off-site: child and adolescent psychiatrist
Medical record and communication	Usually shared EMR plus in-person communication	Medical records kept separate Mental health team is remote and accessible via hotline Outpatient psychiatric evaluation reports sent to PPCP	Shared EMR for on-site behavioral health clinician/care manager Use of clinical registry for tracking patient progress and measures
Advantages in practice	Behavioral health clinician role highly flexible Carefully coordinated referrals ("warm hand-offs")	Consultation primarily conducted by child and adolescent psychiatrists Immediate telephone consultation Scalable across a large population	Use of clinical measures for tracking, clinical feedback, and accountability Strongest evidence base
Challenges in practice	Usually not staffed by child and adolescent psychiatrists, therefore PPCP not provided with psychopharmacologic treatment recommendations Difficulty funding indirect (nonbillable) services	Service offered on-demand: requires primary care provider to recognize the need for consultation; engagement varies widely across practices	Variable insurance coverage for pediatric care Requires higher ratios of embedded behavioral health clinicians in relation to panel size when compared with BHC model

Abbreviation: EMC, electronic medical record.

adolescent psychiatry workforce to the primary care workforce, with an associated shift in the role of the child and adolescent psychiatrist from directly treating patients to serving as a consultant or trainer. The integrated/collaborative care model is most appropriate for delivering mental health treatment from the pediatric primary care team to patients with mild to moderate severity and complexity. Conversely, PPCPs refer patients with more severe and complex conditions to a child and adolescent psychiatrist for treatment and management. In this situation, the PPCP maintains communication with the child and adolescent psychiatrist about these patients' mental health treatment and provides consultation regarding relevant physical health issues.

Despite the myriad advantages, there are significant challenges to integrating the delivery of mental health services into pediatric primary care. These include the relative lack of training and preparation for pediatric providers in child psychiatry,[10] inadequate funding, administrative barriers,[11] and shortages of space and time in modern primary care settings. These institutional constraints have the potential to generate moral distress in which the PPCPs and the child and adolescent psychiatrists who participate in these models must act in a manner contrary to their personal and professional values. Considering these challenges, the practice of integrated/collaborative care in the pediatric primary care setting necessitates careful ethical analysis.

ETHICAL CONSIDERATIONS
Social Justice

The ethical value of social justice in health care is defined as the fair and equitable distribution of goods in society. In light of the identified gap between the need for pediatric mental health care and the significant and ongoing shortage of child and adolescent psychiatrists, taking a population health perspective informs our thinking of how best to use the limited resources we have to ensure social justice and enhance the well-being of children.

Integrated/collaborative care models for pediatric mental health care may be viewed as a form of resource allocation. Rationing refers to situations of absolute scarcity, whereas the term resource allocation is reserved for relative scarcity. Resource allocation has been defined as "to regulate, through explicit or implicit means, access to beneficial healthcare under conditions of relative scarcity."[12] To the authors' knowledge, integrated/collaborative care models have not been explicitly labeled as a form of resource allocation, although they argue this consideration is a useful framework given the ethical implications. The relevant moral principles embedded in the 3 philosophic theories of utilitarianism, deontology, and political liberalism are used to aid in our ethical analysis of social justice within integrated/collaborative care models (**Table 2**).

Utilitarianism

John Stuart Mill was a nineteenth century British philosopher who extended the work of Jeremy Bentham and developed the key principles of the ethical theory of utilitarianism. In utilitarianism, the value of an action (ie, the action's moral worth) derives entirely from the action's consequences or outcomes. As such, utilitarianism is a consequentialist theory in which the end result can justify the means used to obtain the result. Mill defined an action as morally right in proportion to maximizing happiness and morally wrong if the action should result in the opposite outcome. Mill's principle became known as the *Greatest Happiness Principle*, which translates into the greatest good for the greatest number.[13] Justice is anchored in the principle of utility, which strives to produce the maximum balance of positive value over negative value.[14]

Applying the principle of distributive justice embedded in utilitarianism may cause unintended negative consequences for individuals or groups of people. Although challenges to utilitarianism's concept of justice exist, the theory has been successful in promoting just health policies that embrace resource allocation and cost-effectiveness analysis.[15] Overall, a utilitarian view of justice supports an integrated/collaborative care model for mental health care, as its innate design aims to maximize care for a greater number of children.

Deontology

The German Enlightenment philosopher Immanuel Kant developed a theory of morality known as the deontological theory. In deontology, an action is determined morally permissible if an individual is acting from their ethical obligation or duty. This construct sharply contrasts with utilitarianism's determination grounded on consequences and the greatest benefit.[16] Kant's *Formula of Humanity* underscores that all individuals have equal moral standing and are deserving of respect.[17] Although utilitarian

Table 2
Ethical analysis of justice within integrated/collaborative care models

Philosophic Theory	Articulated by	Key Principles and Concept of Justice	Support for Integrated/ Collaborative Care Models?
Utilitarianism	Jeremy Bentham (1748–1832) and John Stuart Mill (1806–1873)	Consequentialist theory: value (moral worth) of an action derives entirely from its consequences (outcomes) Mill's *Greatest Happiness Principle*: the greatest good for the greatest number Mill viewed distributive justice as grounded in the principle of utility Obligations of justice typically establish associated rights for individuals that should be enforced by law	Yes Supports just health policies, congruent with cost-benefit analysis Integrated/collaborative care models by design serve to maximize mental health care for a greater number of children
Deontology	Immanuel Kant (1724–1804)	Greek *deontos:* what must be done; duty Actions are right or wrong based on the obligations or duties we have to each other *Formula of Humanity*: all beings have infinite worth, equal moral standing, and deserve respect *Categorical Imperative*: act in a way that your action could become a universal law of nature Conflicts with paradigm of resource allocation	No Views each human being as having moral worth Unlike utilitarianism, deontology does not endorse the end justifying the means Ethical principles and duties derived from deontology are prominent in codes of health care ethics

(continued on next page)

Table 2
(continued)

Philosophic Theory	Articulated by	Key Principles and Concept of Justice	Support for Integrated/ Collaborative Care Models?
Political Liberalism	John Rawls (1921–2002) Norman Daniels (1942-)	*Justice as fairness theory*: comprehensive view, citizens are free and equal, society should be fair *Liberty Principle*: rights to basic political liberties (freedom of speech, assembly, religion, due process) *Fair Equality of Opportunity*: elected office and careers should be open to all, fair opportunity for disadvantaged to move ahead in society *Difference Principle:* permissible for unequal distribution of basic social and economic goods, but only if the inequality benefits the least advantaged Daniels extended the tenants of Rawls' theory of *Fair Equality of Opportunity* to health care Health care needs are special; disease and disability restrict an individual's range of opportunities Societal obligation to reduce barriers to fair equality of opportunities such as health care Health care systems, policies, and allocation of resources should be designed to guarantee justice through fair equality of opportunity	Yes Norman Daniels' extension of John Rawls' theory supports integrated/ collaborative care models of care, as it aims to meet the mental health care needs of more children, congruent with the principle of equality of opportunity

principles can be understood as the end justifies the means, Kant's writing is clearly otherwise: act so that you use humanity, as much in your person as in the person of every other, always at the same time as an end and never merely as a means.[17] Kant further proposed the *Categorical Imperative*: act in a way such that your action could become a universal law of nature.[17] As a philosophic theory, deontology is concerned with moral duties acted on by individuals and is not designed to guide public health policy or health care systems. The essence of the humanity principle conflicts with the paradigm of resource allocation. Thus, a deontological perspective does not support an integrated/collaborative care model. Ethical principles and duties derived from deontology are incorporated into codes of health care ethics and are discussed later with respect to ethical guidance for the integrated/collaborative care team.

Political liberalism

John Rawls's political liberalism theory articulated justice as fairness in what he called the principle of *Fair Equality of Opportunity*.[18] Rawls focused on the right to basic liberties (the *Liberty Principle*) and identified that inequalities in the distribution of social primary goods (ie, income, rights, and opportunities) are permissible, but only if the inequality benefits the least advantaged (the *Difference Principle*).[18] Rawls did not include health care among social primary goods, nor did he extend the implications of his theory into health care policy.

Norman Daniels work expanded on Rawls's principles of justice and applied them to health care systems. Daniels explains the connection between health care and social justice as follows, "The central moral importance, for purposes of justice, of preventing disease and disability (construed broadly to include public health and environmental measures as personal medical services) derives from the way in which protecting normal functioning contributes to protecting opportunities."[19] Daniels identifies a societal duty to design and implement health care systems that reduce barriers and promote the allocation of health care resources through fair equality of opportunity[20] It is argued that an integrated/collaborative care model aligns with egalitarian concepts of social justice by extending access to mental health care for children and thereby increasing the range of opportunities for children.

Additional concerns

Other important ethical considerations of social justice deserve our attention. Those with power and privilege are able to access direct child psychiatric services. Geographic location, lack of and type of insurance, language and communication barriers, and perceived stigma contribute to reduced use of mental health services. In the United States, the distribution of direct care versus indirect care is not determined by a triage system in which the most severe or complex cases receive direct care. Social determinants of health including (but not limited to) income inequality, unemployment, adverse childhood experiences, food insecurity, discrimination, and toxic neighborhood environments are key contributors in the development, severity, and persistence of mental illness and substance use disorders. Social determinants of health can also lead to, or worsen, barriers to access and the receipt of child mental health services.

Integrated/collaborative care models are not a substitute for public policies, laws, and structural changes that promote social justice. However, practicing within an integrated/collaborative care model offers increased access and familiarity and can be less stigmatizing to those who have already experienced discrimination. Furthermore, programmatic innovations and targeted strategies in integrated/collaborative care models for pediatric mental health care may offer opportunities to address problems of health equity in clinical populations.

Informed Consent

Informed consent is defined as providing the patient and the parent/guardian information about the proposed treatment, risks and benefits of treatment, alternative treatment options, and the likely course of the clinical condition in the absence of treatment. Within an integrated/collaborative care model, informed consent ensures transparency by providing information about the model itself and should precede any discussion regarding informed consent for a specific treatment intervention. Runyan and colleagues[21] write, "True informed consent requires a patient centered conversation at an appropriate level of health literacy and cultural competency, including a discussion of potential implications of a shared medical record, of a BHC seeing multiple family members, and similar scenarios." Informed consent is a process that promotes discussion and provides an opportunity to ask questions. The pediatric patient should receive information about the integrated/collaborative care model according to their developmental capacity for understanding the implications to their care. Parents/guardians are the decision makers for the type of care their child will receive. PPCPs should offer parents/guardians treatment alternatives, including the option to decline integrated/collaborative care services, and when appropriate provide referral information.

Minor children generally require parental/guardian consent before medical care. However, each state determines the statutes for the rights of minors to consent to health care. Minors who are considered "a mature minor" and who qualify as "an emancipated minor" (legally free of parental/guardian control) can also consent or refuse treatment. There are exceptions that allow adolescents, who may otherwise delay or forgo care, to receive treatment without parental/guardian consent, such as treatment of sexually transmitted infections, or for contraceptive services. Furthermore, the age when minors may consent for mental health care or psychotropic medications varies between states and depends on the level of care received—outpatient versus inpatient. Clinicians working within an integrated/collaborative care model need to be familiar with their state statutes and mental health regulations. It is critical to have policies and procedures in place for addressing issues of parental/guardian and minor consent when care shifts from physical health care to encompassing behavioral health care.

A member (or members) of the integrated/collaborative care team may become aware of highly sensitive information, including information that raises concern for the risks of life-threatening, abusive, or otherwise harmful behaviors. From the start, the PPCP should inform pediatric patients and parents/guardians what information will remain confidential versus what information must be shared. Providers may not keep information relevant to mandated reporting and other safety concerns confidential. The integrated/collaborative care team should establish a clear policy outlining the degree of confidentiality upheld. This policy must be consistent with individual state laws delineating the degree of disclosure to parents/guardians that is permitted and/or required. Information sharing and consultation within an integrated/collaborative care model raises ethical issues of privacy, confidentiality, autonomy (of both the parent/guardian and the pediatric patient), scope of practice, beneficence, and nonmaleficence.

Federal and state regulations have placed a higher level of protection for mental health care and substance use treatment records compared with other medical records. Integrated/collaborative care practices will need to address how accessible this information is to colleagues and consultants in electronic medical records. In some states, permission to release records resides with the individual who consents to the treatment.

The Principles of Proportionate Reason

Richard McCormick's 3-fold criteria of proportionate reason is used to evaluate the moral integrity of integrated/collaborative care models within a normative ethical framework. The principles of proportionate reason determine objectively and concretely the rightness and wrongness of actions. Weighing an action's effect on all ends and values must occur before a moral assessment of the action's proportionality. A final decision can be made after all moral values have been considered and compared—within the context of a particular culture, with a particular history, with a particular experience—to be proportionate or disproportionate. Proportionality is always the criterion where actions have the potential to cause damage. The integrated/collaborative care model for pediatric mental health care, as all imperfect things in medicine, has the potential for individual and social damage. The sense of what individuals ought to do is thus informed by past experience and uncertainty with regard to future behavior and its long-term effects.[21]

For McCormick, proportionate reason for permitting the occurrence of potential harm (otherwise judged as prohibited within a normative moral calculus) signifies 3 things: (1) the value at stake is at least equal to the value being sacrificed; (2) there is no less harmful way, here and now, to protect the value; and (3) the means used to protect the value, here and now, will not undermine the value in the long run.[20] Conversely, an action is disproportionate if (1) a lesser value is preferred to a more important one; (2) harm is unnecessarily caused in the protection of a greater good; or (3) in the circumstances, the manner of protecting the good, here and now, will undermine the good in the long run.[20] To determine if an action involving potential harm is proportionate, one must judge whether the specific choice is the best possible service to all values in the difficult and imperfect circumstances. The best promotion of all values will depend on how one defines and understands the circumstances. An adequate account of the circumstances must include not simply how much quantitative good can be salvaged from conflicting values but also the weight and balance of social implications and reverberating aftereffects (insofar as they can be foreseen). This account will test generalizability, consider cultural climate, draw from historical wisdom, seek guidance from others, and distance itself from self-interested tendencies.

Before applying McCormick's *first criterion* of proportionality (the value at stake is at least equal to the value being sacrificed) to the action of implementing integrated/collaborative care models for pediatric mental health care, it is necessary to first identify both the value at stake and the value being sacrificed. This paper defines the value at stake as the patient's individual and social mental health, well-being, and safety—elements that together comprise the patient's ability to seek, identify, and act on the good.[21] This paper defines the value being sacrificed as the patient's experience of a traditional, comprehensive model of psychiatric care, involving a direct, robust psychiatrist-patient relationship. Applied in the current context, the first criterion thus becomes: is the pediatric patient's individual and social mental health, well-being, and safety at least equal to the patient's experience of a traditional, comprehensive model for psychiatric care, involving a direct, robust psychiatrist-patient relationship? Given the scarcity of pediatric psychiatrists, the high likelihood of children having little or no access to needed psychiatric care makes the patient's individual and social mental health, well-being, and safety substantially more vulnerable. For this reason alone, one can conclude that access to some psychiatric treatment is of equal, if not greater, value to having imperfect access (or likely no access at all). In this way, integrated/collaborative care models for pediatric mental health care meet McCormick's first criterion of proportionality. Indeed, the value at stake is at least equal to the value being scarified.

McCormick's *second criterion* of proportionality requires that there exists no less harmful way, here and now, to protect the value at stake.[20] Applied in the current context, the second criterion thus becomes: does there exist a no less harmful way, here and now, to protect the pediatric patient's individual and social mental health, well-being, and safety than to facilitate access to integrated/collaborative care models in circumstances for which access to traditional models is not, and perhaps may never be, possible for the patient? Given the gravity of untreated psychosocial conditions on the patient's individual and social mental health, well-being, and safety, it is reasonable to conclude that facilitating access to these models is the least harmful and perhaps a harmless, means to secure the value at stake. In this way, integrated/collaborative care models for pediatric mental health care meet McCormick's second criterion of proportionality. Indeed, there exists no less harmful way, here and now, to protect the value at stake.

McCormick's *third criterion* of proportionality requires that within the circumstances, the means used to achieve the value, here and now, will not undermine the value in the long run.[20] Applied in the current context, the third criterion thus becomes: in circumstances with concern for the pediatric patient's worsening psychosocial condition, and with a known difficulty in accessing traditional models of psychiatric care, do the means of accessing integrated/collaborative care models to protect the value of the patient's individual and social mental health, well-being, and safety undermine the patient's individual and social mental health, well-being, and safety in the long run? Potential counterarguments include the perception that an imperfect model of psychiatric care may in fact be so incomplete as to (1) cooperate in failing to recognize the subtle nuances of life-threatening conditions or (2) discourage the patient from seeking needed psychiatric care in the future. Yet, such a dispute is morally shortsighted insofar as (1) not having access to traditional psychiatric care would guarantee such a failure to recognize the nuances of life-threatening conditions, and (2) the lack of access would actively contribute to the patient's discouragement from seeking psychiatric care in the future. For these among other reasons, integrated/collaborative care models of pediatric psychiatry meet McCormick's third criterion of proportionality. Indeed, in this circumstance, the means used to achieve the value, here and now, does not undermine (but rather overall enhances) the value in the long run.

Ethical Responsibility Within an Imperfect Model

Guidance at the integrated/collaborative care team level

Integrated/collaborative care models innately include multidisciplinary professionals, each guided by their own profession's code of ethics. The very act of delivering team-based interprofessional care will inevitably create conflicts between different guild-specific ethical guidelines. Deontological principles focus on one's duties and obligations and are widely applied to biomedical ethics and incorporated universally into health care codes of ethics. Different professional codes of health care ethics share common ethical principles such as autonomy, beneficence, nonmaleficence, and justice. Yet, what may present as an ethical dilemma for a behavioral health provider may not be an issue for a primary care provider. Runyan and colleagues discuss common ethical dilemmas in collaborative care and propose shared interprofessional principles to address these challenges.[19] The ethical guidance for the collaborative care model is grounded on 4 principles: (1) help/do no harm—a combination of beneficence and nonmaleficence that prompts clinicians to be explicit about practice decisions; (2) patient-centered informed consent for the model of care; (3) transparent consultation with colleagues and patients; and (4) transparent documentation. These principles are complementary to guild-specific ethics and are set forth to resolve ethical issues.

Support for interprofessional ethical guidance continues to evolve. Thus, some investigators recommend practicing close to one's own ethical code until clear ethical guidance is established. Although others such as Kanzler and colleagues[22] present a stepped process to address differences in ethical codes, Runyan and colleagues[23] support determining the root cause of the problem. A specific clinical and ethical challenge unique to the model is present when a patient's clinical needs exceed the limits of what can be provided in the collaborative care model. In this situation, the team should make recommendations to benefit the patient, be clear about the limitations of collaborative care, and facilitate transfer of care.

Guidance for individual members within an integrated/collaborative care team

The American Medical Association Code of Medical Ethics Opinion 10.8 addresses effective physician leadership for collaborative care. Physicians are expected to model ethical leadership by appreciating the limits of their own and other team members' skills and expertise, understanding their role in the patient's care, providing clarity on individual responsibilities and accountability, being open to implementing insights from other team members, and demonstrating teamwork skills. The goal is to "encourage open discussion of ethical and clinical concerns and foster a team culture in which each member's opinion is heard and considered and team members share accountability for decisions and outcomes."[24]

Integrated/collaborative care models deliver team-based care that is vastly different from providing one-on-one care. Training, orientation, and understanding interprofessional models of health care delivery will enhance the capabilities of clinicians without prior experience working within this model. The Substance Abuse and Mental Health Services Administration—Health Resources and Services Administration Center for Integrated Health Solutions offers core competencies for the collaborative care model that are relevant to both the primary care and behavioral health workforces. The 9 core competencies are (1) interpersonal communication; (2) collaboration and teamwork; (3) screening and assessment; (4) care planning and care coordination; (5) intervention; (6) cultural competence and adaptation; (7) systems-oriented practice; (8) practice-based learning and quality improvement; and (9) informatics.[25] The core competencies for collaborative care establish a framework to deliver quality care within the model and identify practice standards to guide all team members.

Ethical tensions between the parent/guardian, pediatric patient, and the integrated/collaborative care team

Children depend on their parent/guardian to recognize their mental health problems and to seek help on their behalf.[26] Parental/guardian and patient engagement with the integrated/collaborative care team is predicated on their trust in the PPCP's ability to deliver high-quality mental health care. Ethical dilemmas that arise at the interface of the parent/guardian and pediatric patient within an integrated/collaborative care model have received little attention in the literature.

For example, one can envision a situation in which a parent who previously consented to a collaborative care model now wishes to exercise their parental autonomy, as they believe receiving mental health care from their PPCP is no longer in the best interest of their child and insists the consulting child psychiatrist directly treat their child. The PPCP and the team's engagement with the parent deteriorates; however, the pediatric patient is pleased with the care and wants to continue. This scenario highlights several ethical principles: parental autonomy versus child autonomy, the collaborative team's obligations to both the parent/guardian and the pediatric patient, beneficence versus nonmaleficence, fidelity to the model, and ensuring best practices within the model. The response of the collaborative care team can draw on their established processes and shared interprofessional ethical guidance to address such dilemmas.

In another situation, the pediatric patient's mental illness may progress to a more serious condition (eg, mania or early onset psychosis) beyond the competency of the PPCP. The recommendation for inpatient mental health treatment may not be acceptable to the parent or even to all members of the team. Team members may question the parent's decisional capacity or perhaps raise the question of medical neglect. Other team members may feel it is the parent's right to start a trial of medication at home. The consulting child psychiatrist advocates for hospitalization and expresses a priority for honoring the best interest standard of the child. The PPCP supports the parent's desire to treat at home, consistent with the standard of constrained parental autonomy. These challenging treatment situations can be approached with guidance for the collaborative care team and individual members of the team, as outlined earlier.

CLINICAL CASE

Henry, a 16-year-old boy with a longstanding history of ADHD, presented to Dr Jones, his primary care provider from birth, with a 3-month history of worsening depressed mood, withdrawal from family, academic failure, difficulty sleeping, loss of energy, and habitual use of marijuana. He denied any current or past history of suicidal ideation nor self-injurious behavior. Before the onset of these symptoms, his parents had become separated and he experienced a painful breakup with his girlfriend. Dr Jones decided to proceed with evaluating and treating this patient with the support of consultation and care coordination from his regional CPAP. He contacted the CPAP hotline and discussed the case with the child and adolescent psychiatrist who was on duty. An avid user of the CPAP, Dr Jones, had cultivated strong collegial relationships with the members of the CPAP team and had grown increasingly comfortable evaluating and managing patients with mild to moderate depression. After the telephone consultation, Dr Jones referred Henry to a local outpatient therapist and initiated a trial of fluoxetine to be added to the methylphenidate that he had been prescribing for the past 5 years. Despite the absence of current suicidal ideation, the consulting child and adolescent psychiatrist recommended that Dr Jones develop a safety plan with Henry, should suicidal ideation emerge in the coming weeks.

Dr Jones saw the patient for follow-up 2 weeks after his initial visit. At that time, Henry was tolerating the medication well, and his initial appointment with the therapist was scheduled for the following week. At 4 weeks, Henry reported a positive first encounter with the therapist and subtle improvement in depressive symptoms. At both visits, the patient continued to deny suicidal ideation. Subsequently, Henry missed his next follow-up appointment 4 weeks later. Approximately 12 weeks after his initial appointment, Dr Jones received a call from the parent after Henry was admitted to the pediatric intensive care unit following an intentional overdose of acetaminophen. Dr Jones learned Henry had stopped taking his fluoxetine, dropped out of therapy, and was caught cheating on an examination just before the overdose. Although Henry was in stable condition, Dr Jones experienced moral distress, feeling that he had let Henry down, and questioned if the patient would have been better served under the direct care of a child and adolescent psychiatrist.

DISCUSSION

Participation in an integrated/collaborative care model offers many advantages. However, as is the general practice of medicine, an integrated/collaborative care model is an imperfect science, and therefore, it is imperative to recognize and understand ethical considerations within its practice. The challenges inherent in the model can produce moral distress among those involved. Moral distress is the inability to act in accord with one's own individual and professional ethical core values and perceived obligations due to internal and external (institutional and/or societal) constraints.[27,28] It is important to acknowledge and examine moral distress, as research identifies this

Table 3			
Applying McCormick's principles of proportionate reason			
Principle Criterion	**Criterion Description**	**Specified Question**	**Applied Conclusion**
First	The value at stake is at least equal to the value being sacrificed.	Is the pediatric patient's individual and social mental health, well-being, and safety at least equal to the patient's experience of a traditional model for direct care by a psychiatrist?	Henry's immediate access to psychiatric care provided by Dr Jones under the direction of the CPAP consultant is at least equal to the sacrificed value of delayed access to direct care by a psychiatrist.
Second	There exists no less harmful way, here and now, to protect the value at stake.	Does there exist no less harmful way, here and now, to protect the pediatric patient's individual and social mental health, well-being, and safety than to facilitate access to integrated/collaborative care models in circumstances for which access to traditional models is not, and perhaps may never be, possible for the patient?	Obtaining psychiatric care provided by Dr Jones under the direction of the CPAP consultant is, here and now, the least harmful of the imperfect options.
Third	In the circumstances, the means used to achieve the value, here and now, will not undermine the value in the long run.	In circumstances, with concern for the pediatric patient's worsening psychosocial condition, and with a known difficulty in accessing traditional models of psychiatric care, do the means of accessing integrated/collaborative care models to protect the value of the patient's individual and social mental health, well-being, and safety undermine the patient's individual and social mental health, well-being, and safety in the long run?	Because of the urgency to treat Henry's progression of symptoms over the preceding 3 months, and the difficulty of accessing traditional models of psychiatric care, having Dr Jones treat Henry under the direction of the CPAP consultant, here and now (vs delayed or no treatment), will not undermine his mental health in the long run.

problem as a leading cause of physician burnout[27] and further may negatively affect a physician's ability to care for patients.

Political liberalism and utilitarianism support the allocation of health care resources by decreasing barriers and thus maximizing the number of individuals receiving behavioral health services. Henry was immediately able to see his PPCP 3 times in a 4-week period. Given the shortage of child and adolescent psychiatrists, it can be inferred Henry's care would have been delayed in a traditional care model. On the other hand, deontological theory questions if Henry received the best possible care and if an extensively trained child and adolescent psychiatrist would have been better suited to appreciate the nuances of Henry's presentation. Unfortunately, bad outcomes occur even with the highest level of care provided by psychiatric experts. Evaluating the application of informed consent, one will question if the parents and patient understood the implications of the CPAP model and if they had been offered the alternative to pursue direct care from a child and adolescent psychiatrist.

McCormick's 3-fold criteria of proportionate reason determines if the potential for harm attributable to Dr Jones providing care in the CPAP model is ethically permissible (**Table 3**). *First*, Henry's immediate access to psychiatric care provided by Dr Jones is at least equal to the value of having delayed access to direct psychiatric care produced by barriers to access. In other words, the value of Henry's mental health is at least equal to the sacrificed value of traditional direct care from a psychiatrist. *Second*, obtaining psychiatric care provided by Dr Jones under the direction of the CPAP consultant may be viewed as the least harmful of the imperfect options. *Third*, because of the urgency to treat Henry's progression of mental health symptoms over the preceding 3 months, and the difficulty of accessing traditional models of psychiatric care, having Dr Jones treat Henry here and now (vs delayed or no treatment) will not undermine his mental health in the long run.

Dr Jones demonstrated beneficence, consideration, and professionalism by seeking immediate consultation, starting an antidepressant, referring for psychotherapy, and scheduling subsequent follow-up—all consistent with clinical practice guidelines. There are several unknowns in this case, including the following: if Dr Jones discussed with Henry and his parents the risk of suicidality and antidepressants; if Dr Jones reviewed symptoms that would escalate safety concerns; if Dr Jones adhered to his primary care practice's protocol for outreach following missed appointments; and if Dr Jones developed a robust crisis plan. The specific issues raised in this case bridge ethical and clinical considerations and are not unique to the CPAP model—or any other integrated/collaborative care model—as they could have likewise presented within the framework of direct psychiatric care.

SUMMARY

The serious and ongoing shortage of child and adolescent psychiatrists limits access to mental health care in the pediatric population. Integrated/collaborative care models have been established to address this problem. Careful analysis of ethical considerations in the practice of integrated/collaborative care in the pediatric primary care setting is vital to protecting the social and emotional well-being and safety of children and adolescents with mental illness. Similar to the general practice of medicine, an integrated/collaborative care model is an imperfect science with its own set of challenges and disadvantages that have the potential to produce moral distress among those involved. Inversely, ethical evaluation supports the use of integrated/collaborative care models, and recent research has demonstrated the advantages and benefits associated with their implementation.

CLINICS CARE POINTS

- A widespread shortage of child and adolescent psychiatrists has led to the development of clinical models for incorporating mental health treatment into primary care. Three models have become most prevalent and include the Behavioral Health Consultant model, Child Psychiatry Access Program model, and Collaborative Care model.

- Integrated/collaborative care models embrace the ethical principle of social justice—identified as a form of resource allocation—and can be further examined through the philosophic constructs of utilitarianism, deontology, and political liberalism to provide ethical guidance.

- Informed consent within an integrated/collaborative care model emphasizes the importance of transparency, presentation of alternatives with the option to decline the model, policies to address consent, and respect for confidentiality within the unique confines of collaboration.

- Richard McCormick's 3-fold model of proportionate reason endorses the ethical permissibility of the potential for harm to the pediatric patient when using an integrated/collaborative care model in place of a traditional model of direct care by a psychiatrist.

- Ethical guidance is offered regarding responsibility at the level of the care team, individual members within the team, and in the context of parental/guardian and child autonomy.

DISCLOSURE

The authors have nothing to disclose.

REFERENCES

1. Whitney DG, Peterson MD. US national and state-level prevalence of mental health disorders and disparities of mental health care use in children. JAMA Pediatr 2019;173(4):389–91.
2. McBain RK, Kofner A, Stein BD, et al. Growth and distribution of child psychiatrists in the United States: 2007-2016. Pediatrics 2019;144(6):e20191576.
3. Committee on Psychosocial Aspects of Child and Family Health and Task Force on Mental Health. Policy statement–The future of pediatrics: mental health competencies for pediatric primary care. Pediatrics 2009;124(1):410–21.
4. Gunn WB Jr, Blount A. Primary care mental health: a new frontier for psychology. J Clin Psychol 2009;65(3):235–52.
5. Sarvet B, Gold J, Bostic JQ, et al. Improving access to mental health care for children: the Massachusetts Child Psychiatry Access Project. Pediatrics 2010; 126(6):1191–200.
6. Raney LE. Integrating primary care and behavioral health: the role of the psychiatrist in the collaborative care model. Am J Psychiatry 2015;172(8):721–8.
7. Asarnow JR, Rozenman M, Wiblin J, et al. Integrated medical-behavioral care compared with usual primary care for child and adolescent behavioral health: a meta-analysis. JAMA Pediatr 2015;169(10):929–37.
8. Stein BD, Kofner A, Vogt WB, et al. A national examination of child psychiatric telephone consultation programs' impact on Children's mental health care utilization. J Am Acad Child Adolesc Psychiatry 2019;58(10):1016–9.
9. Cama S, Knee A, Sarvet B. Impact of child psychiatry access programs on mental health care in pediatric primary care: measuring the parent experience. Psychiatr Serv 2020;71(1):43–8.

10. McMillan JA, Land M Jr, Leslie LK. Pediatric residency education and the behavioral and mental health crisis: a call to action. Pediatrics 2017;139(1):e20162141.
11. American Academy of Child and Adolescent Psychiatry Committee on Health Care Access and Economics Task Force on Mental Health. Improving mental health services in primary care: reducing administrative and financial barriers to access and collaboration. Pediatrics 2009;123(4):1248–51.
12. Emanuel E, Steinmetz A, Schmidt H. Rationing and resource allocation in healthcare essential readings. New York, NY: Oxford University Press; 2018. p. 16.
13. Mill JS. Utilitarianism, liberty and representative government. London, England: J. M. Dent & Sons; 1910. p. 5–24.
14. Mill JS. The collected works of john Stuart Mill, vol. 10. Toronto: University of Toronto Press; 1969. Chapter 5.
15. Beauchamp TL, Childress JF. Principles of biomedical ethics. 7th edition. New York, NY: Oxford University Press; 2013. p. 255.
16. Emanuel E, Steinmetz A, Schmidt H. Rationing and resource allocation in healthcare essential readings. New York, NY: Oxford University Press; 2018. p. 37.
17. Johnson R, Cureton A. Kant's moral philosophy. Stanford Encyclopedia of philosophy. 2019. Available at: https://plato.stanford.edu/archives/spr2019/entries/kant-moral/. Accessed March 1, 2021.
18. Rawls J. A theory of justice. Rev edition. Cambridge, MA: Harvard University Press; 1999. p. 52–8.
19. Daniels N. Justice, health, and healthcare. Am J Bioeth 2001;1(2):2–16.
20. Daniels N. Just health care. New York, NY: Cambridge University Press; 1985. p. 34–58.
21. Runyan CN, Carter-Henry S, Ogbeide S. Ethical challenges unique to the primary care behavioral health (PCBH) model. J Clin Psychol Med Settings 2018;25(2):224–36.
22. Kanzler KE, Goodie JL, Hunter CL, et al. From colleague to patient: ethical challenges in integrated primary care. Fam Syst Health 2013;31(1):41–8.
23. Runyan C, Robinson P, Gould DA. Ethical issues facing providers in collaborative primary care settings: do current guidelines suffice to guide the future of team based primary care? Fam Syst Health 2013;31(1):1–8.
24. Code of medical ethics opinion 10.8. American medical association. Available at: https://www.ama-assn.org/delivering-care/ethics/collaborative-care. Accessed February 1, 2021.
25. Hodge MA, Moris JA, Laraia M, et al. Core competencies for integrated behavioral health and primary care. Washington, DC: SAMHSA – HRSA Center for Integrated Health Solutions; 2014.
26. Sayal K, Tischler V, Coope C, et al. Parental help-seeking in primary care for child and adolescent mental health concerns: qualitative study. Br J Psychiatry 2010;197(6):476–81.
27. Fumis RRL, Junqueira Amarante GA, de Fátima Nascimento A, et al. Moral distress and its contribution to the development of burnout syndrome among critical care providers. Ann Intensive Care 2017;7(1):71.
28. Dzeng E, Wachter RM. Ethics in conflict: moral distress as a root cause of burnout. J Gen Intern Med 2020;35(2):409–11.

Interprofessional Education in Child and Adolescent Mental Health: A Scoping Review

Michelle Kiger, Maj, USAF, MC[a,b,]*,
Kara Knickerbocker, DO, Capt, USAF, MC[b],
Caitlin Hammond, MD, Maj, USAF, MC[a,b], Suzie C. Nelson, MD[a,b]

KEYWORDS

- Adolescent mental health • Child mental health • Interprofessional education
- Interprofessional training • Scoping review

KEY POINTS

- Interprofessional education (IPE) in child and adolescent mental health (CAMH) is endorsed by multiple professional organizations
- IPE interventions in CAMH can involve a wide range of medical, mental health, allied health, educational, and community-based professionals
- Learners report overwhelmingly positive perceptions of and attitudes toward IPE following participation in IPE interventions
- Evidence for behavioral, patient-level, and systems-level outcomes tied to CAMH IPE is positive but less robust than for attitudinal and knowledge-based outcomes
- Future CAMH IPE interventions should consider employing practice-based delivery methods and seek higher-level educational outcomes

Abbreviations	
ADHD	Attention-deficit-hyperactivity disorder
BART	Biofeedback-assisted relaxation training
CAMH	Child and adolescent mental health
IDP	[Interaction with Disabled Persons
IPE	Interprofessional education
IPEC	Interprofessional Education Collaborative
ISVS	Interprofessional socialization and valuing scale
RIPLS	Readiness for interprofessional learning scale
WHO	World Health Organization

[a] Uniformed Services University of the Health Sciences, Bethesda, MD, USA; [b] Wright-Patterson Medical Center, 4881 Sugar Maple Drive, Dayton, OH 45433, USA
* Corresponding author. Wright-Patterson Medical Center, 4881 Sugar Maple Drive, Dayton, OH 45433, USA
E-mail address: michelle.e.kiger@gmail.com

Child Adolesc Psychiatric Clin N Am 30 (2021) 713–726
https://doi.org/10.1016/j.chc.2021.07.001
1056-4993/21/© 2021 Elsevier Inc. All rights reserved.
childpsych.theclinics.com

INTRODUCTION

Caring for children with behavioral and mental health concerns is a common, yet often complex, endeavor for physicians, educators, and a range of mental health professionals. While each of these specialties brings particular expertise to the provision of care for these children, achieving integrated, interprofessional care delivery remains an elusive goal in many settings.[1,2] Inadequate knowledge or training in mental health care or collaboration,[3–5] divergent approaches to patient care, differences in professional cultures, professional role ambiguity, and lack of teamwork can all pose significant barriers to interprofessional practice.[1,2,6] Despite these challenges, a wide range of professional organizations have strongly advocated for interprofessional mental health care delivery, including the World Health Organization (WHO),[7] American Academy of Pediatrics,[8] and the American Academy of Child and Adolescent Psychiatry.[9] Therefore, in order to prepare clinicians for interprofessional practice, many have called for increased interprofessional education (IPE)—defined by the WHO as "students from two or more professions learn[ing] about, from and with each other to enable effective collaboration and improve health outcomes."[7] IPE has been demonstrated to improve integrated health care delivery, thereby strengthening health systems and improving patient outcomes.[7] However, little is known about the scope, characteristics, and effectiveness of IPE within child and adolescent mental health (CAMH) care in order to guide IPE efforts.

Most prior studies examining mental health IPE have focused on adults, although even this literature is limited in scope. A recent systematic review of the effects of mental health IPE by Marcussen and colleagues[6] identified eight studies and found generally positive effects of IPE on practitioner attitudes toward other disciplines, knowledge gains, and collaborative skills; evidence demonstrating changes in behavior or practice was lacking. However, their search criteria targeted mental health conditions in adults, and they only included studies involving undergraduate-level students. Similarly, a scoping literature review by Landoll and colleagues[10] focused on IPE within primary care behavioral health and reported improvements in learner perceptions, knowledge, and attitudes from such interventions, but only three of the 21 included studies involved pediatrics. IPE on substance use[11] and dementia[12] has also received much attention with mostly positive learner perceptions and learning outcomes.

These prior studies offer a starting point for examining IPE within CAMH, but it is difficult to extrapolate findings from adult-focused mental health education to pediatrics. First, the adult literature on IPE has generally not examined mental health topics more specific to pediatrics, such as attention-deficit-hyperactivity disorder (ADHD), autism, or developmental delays. Furthermore, even for mental health conditions common to both populations, such as anxiety and depression, treatment approaches often differ. Finally, the participants and teachers involved in IPE focused on CAMH can include additional professions that would not likely be included in adult mental health IPE, such as teachers, school counselors, and other community youth workers. IPE interventions specifically within the realm of CAMH have not been reviewed.

In order to effectively equip medical and mental health professionals for interprofessional practice in CAMH, we must identify elements of effective IPE specific to this realm. With this knowledge, educators can build upon prior successful interventions and strive toward attaining higher levels of evidence for future work in IPE. Therefore, we conducted a scoping literature review to examine IPE interventions within CAMH with respect to their participants, educational characteristics, and outcomes.

METHODS

We conducted a scoping review in accordance with Arksey and O'Malley's[13] five-step framework. This method of literature review is appropriate for newer topics that have yet to be explored systematically. Congruent with Arksey and O'Malley's[13] proposed reasons for conducting scoping reviews, our aims were "to examine the extent, range, and nature of research" in the area and "to summarize and disseminate research findings" on CAMH IPE.

Beginning with the first step in the framework, the authors collectively defined three research questions to guide our search:

(1) What learners and teachers have been involved in IPE interventions focusing on CAMH?
(2) What are the characteristics of reported educational interventions within CAMH IPE—including their topics, duration, settings, and educational methods?
(3) What are the outcomes of IPE interventions in CAMH in the literature?

We conducted step two of the framework—identifying relevant studies—by searching four relevant databases: PubMed, Embase, PsychINFO, and Cochrane Databases. With the assistance of a medical librarian, we developed a search strategy in order to capture all relevant studies within the peer-reviewed literature—step 3. After three rounds of iteratively refining the search strategy and repeating the database searches until we could identify no additional relevant studies, our final search strategy used the terms: "Interprofessional OR inter-professional OR interdisciplinary OR inter-disciplinary" AND "Child OR adolescent OR teenage* OR youth" AND "Mental-health OR depression OR depressive disorders OR schizophrenia OR bipolar OR behavioral-health OR mood-disorder* OR anxiet*." We also identified additional relevant articles through hand searches of included manuscripts.

Our criteria for inclusion were that papers must: (1) involve IPE, (2) explicitly address CAMH—exclusively or as part of a broader mental health intervention that also included adult/general mental health, (3) describe an educational intervention, and (4) be published in English. We considered all types of manuscripts for inclusion in our study (ie, original research papers, educational innovation reports/pilot studies, review papers, commentaries, editorials) but only included papers such as commentaries or editorials if they also explicitly described a study or intervention (even if that was not the entire focus of the paper). We limited the search to studies published in 2008 or later due to capture more recent interventions and because an upward inflection point in study publications on CAMH IPE was noted at that date in our database searches. Studies addressing only baseline learner attitudes or perceptions related to IPE without an associated intervention or educational session were excluded. With respect to mental health topics, we included papers covering any aspect of CAMH, including parenting or practice-based interventions in which participants trained together on a range of mental health concerns that presented to the practice. IPE interventions on childhood developmental delays that are not usually treated by mental health professionals (eg, isolated speech/language delay) were excluded. One author (M.K.) screened titles and abstracts from the database searches to eliminate irrelevant papers. The full text of articles that passed the first screening was independently reviewed by two authors to determine final eligibility for inclusion. Disagreements among reviewers were resolved by consensus among the entire team of authors.

In step four of the framework, the authors collectively created a data extraction tool to record data from the included manuscripts. In creating the tool, we were guided by the 3P model forwarded by Reeves and colleagues,[14] which advocates attending to presage (ie, characteristics of learners and environment), process (ie, the conduct of the educational session/intervention), and product (ie, outcome) factors when evaluating IPE interventions. Accordingly, the tool included details of learner and teacher characteristics, educational setting, educational methods, duration of interventions, study methodology, the type of data collected, whether the analysis was informed by a particular educational theory, and findings/outcomes related to IPE. We also classified outcomes according to Kirkpatrick's[15] levels of evaluation: learner perceptions of or reactions to the interventions (Level 1); changes in learner knowledge, skills, or attitudes (Level 2); changes in learner behavior (Level 3); and changes in patient-level or organizational outcomes (Level 4). We further specified whether outcomes reported at Level 3 or 4 were based on learner self-report only (eg, a participant reporting they collaborate more frequently with interprofessional teams after completing an IPE intervention) or based on additional measures (eg, chart reviews, observations). After pilot testing the data extraction tool and making revisions to ensure all relevant information was included, two authors independently completed the final data extraction form (Appendix 1) on each included manuscript.

In the final step—summarizing and reporting results—we collated responses from the data extraction tool into a shared Excel spreadsheet and analyzed data to create final categories for reporting. This step involved deciding on final labels for reporting results within the three categories of the 3P model, tallying the number of studies/interventions that met each reporting criterion, and analyzing results for key commonalities and areas of divergence among interventions. We did not explicitly engage additional stakeholders—an optional sixth step proposed by Arksey and O'Malley (2005)—but in accordance with best practices for scoping reviews as recommended by Levac and colleagues,[16] our author team did include a range of professional backgrounds relevant to the subject area, including two pediatric faculty (M.K., C.H.), a child psychiatrist (S.N.), and a pediatric chief resident (K.K.).

RESULTS

We identified 778 manuscripts through our database searches, with 304 being duplicates (**Fig. 1**). Of the 474 articles screened by title and abstract, 367 were excluded as irrelevant. A full-text review of the remaining 107 articles led to 82 being excluded because they did not involve IPE, did not explicitly address child or adolescent mental health, and/or did not describe an actual intervention. Hand searches identified 7 additional articles that met full inclusion criteria, yielding a total of 32 articles included. Of note, one pair of included manuscripts[17,18] described the same intervention, and an additional set of three manuscripts[19–21] described another single IPE intervention. Therefore, each set/pair of these studies were reported as a single intervention in the findings below, leading to 29 distinct interventions. A description of all included studies appears in Appendix 1.

Participant Characteristics

IPE interventions described in the studies involved a wide range of learners and teachers (**Table 1**). The most common learners included in IPE interventions were psychology students/trainees (n = 13),[17,18,22–33] followed by nurses (n = 11),[19–22,33–40] attending physicians (n = 10),[19–21,27,28,34,35,37–41] resident/trainee physicians (n = 10),[17,18,22,24,27,28,30–32,36,42] and psychologists (n = 10).[19–21,27,28,34,37–41,43] Many studies also included a diverse range of other healthcare or allied health professionals such as social workers (n = 8),[19–21,34–36,38–41] speech (n = 6),[25,34,43–46] or occupational

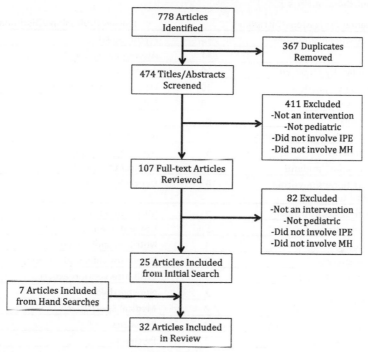

Fig. 1. Prisma diagram of study selection

(n = 7),[19–21,29,34,39,43,45,47] therapists, and behavioral analysts (n = 3).[19–22,28] Interestingly, several studies also included professionals less directly related to the medical or mental health fields, such as teachers/educators (n = 5),[23,25,36,41,43] law enforcement (n = 2),[19–21,41] and a range of other community workers.

Similarly, the teachers or preceptors involved in IPE were most often psychologists (n = 13),[17–21,24,26–29,32,33,38,39,42,48] attending physicians (n = 11),[17,18,24,28,31,32,38,39,41–43,48] and speech (n = 7)[42–48] and occupational therapists (n = 5).[38,39,42,45,47] As with IPE learners, several teachers also came from several non-health-care fields such as school teachers/educators (n = 3)[42,43,48] and even a parent of a child with autism (n = 1).[43] Of studies that included physicians or physicians in training (ie, residents or fellows) as teachers or learners, the medical specialties represented were pediatrics (n = 10),[17,18,22,24,28,31,32,34,36,42] psychiatry (n = 10),[27,30,32–34,39–42,48] neurology (n = 4),[22,28,32,34] family medicine (n = 3),[19–22,28] and genetics (n = 1).[28]

Educational Interventions and Study Characteristics

Educational interventions (**Table 2**) were most commonly conducted in outpatient (n = 13)[17,18,22,24,25,28,29,31,32,35,42,44,47,48] clinical settings. The majority of these clinics were either resident continuity clinics (n = 4)[17,18,24,32] or interdisciplinary autism clinics (n = 4).[22,25,29,42] Many also took place in school-based (n = 10)[23,26,28,30,34,43,45–48] or community-based (n = 9)[19–21,23,36–41] settings, including several that occurred at multiple community sites around a particular geographic area[19–21,36,40] and one that involved a global network of workshops.[41] Most of the interventions involving more diverse, nonmedical participants such as youth services workers, law enforcement, or clergy occurred in such community-based settings. Only two interventions were conducted in inpatient settings.[27,35]

Table 1
Participant characteristics

Learner Professions/Disciplines		Teacher Professions/Disciplines	
Psychology students/trainees	13	Psychologists	13
Nurses	11	Attending/faculty physicians	11
Attending/faculty physicians	10	Speech therapists	7
Resident/trainee physicians	10	Occupational therapists	5
Psychologists	10	Social workers	3
Social workers	8	Teachers/educators	3
Occupational therapists/students	7	Nurses	3
Medical students	6	Behavioral analysts	2
Speech therapists/students	6	Physical therapists	2
Nurse practitioners/physician assistants/students	6	Dental hygienists	1
Social work students/trainees	5	Music therapists	1
Teachers/educators	5	Law enforcement	1
Nursing students	4	Nutritionist/dietician	1
Behavioral analysts	3	Parent (of child with autism)	1
Physical therapists/students	3	Crisis intervention expert	1
Dental hygiene students	2	Not specified	8
Music therapist/students	2	**Medical Specialties**	
Pharmacist/pharmacy students	2	Pediatrics	10
Law enforcement	2	Psychiatry	10
Nutritionists/dieticians	2	Neurology	4
Other	12	Family Medicine	3
		Genetics	1
		Not specified	3

Table 2
Educational and study characteristics

Topic Addressed		Educational Methodology	
Autism	11	Didactic	22
General child mental health	10	Practice-based	14
Anxiety	5	Observation	5
Depression	5	Simulation	3
Eating disorders	4	**Length of Intervention**	
Trauma	3	Single day	5
ADHD	2	Multiday	17
Developmental delay	2	Longitudinal	7
Substance use	2	**Study Setting**	
ODD	1	Outpatient	13
Pain management	1	School-based	10
Study Design		Community-based	9
Mixed methods	15	Inpatient	2
Qualitative	9		
Quantitative	8		

Regarding educational methods, interventions described were most often didactic (n = 22),[17–25,27,28,30,32–34,36–43,47,48] but the majority of these employed interactive, participatory methods such as case-based practice or small group discussions. Practice-based interventions in which learners saw patients together were also common (n = 14).[17,18,23–27,29,30,32,37,42,44,46,48] A minority of interventions involved observational interventions in which learners shadowed one another in their clinical practices (n = 5)[22,23,28,33,44] or interprofessional simulation experiences (n = 3).[31,35,45] The duration of interventions varied widely, ranging from a few hours on a single day (n = 5),[22,27,28,35,45] to multi-day sessions (lasting from 2 days to multiple sessions over a semester; n = 17),[19–21,23,26,29–31,33,34,36,38–41,43,44,46,47] to longitudinal embedding of learners with one another over years of training (n = 7).[17,18,24,25,32,37,42,48]

With respect to mental health topics addressed, autism was covered in over twice as many interventions (n = 11)[22–25,28,29,31,43–46] as any other single topic. The next most frequently covered topics were anxiety (n = 5),[19–21,27,30,32,35] depression (n = 5),[19–21,24,30,32,35] and eating disorders (n = 4).[9,35,37–39,53–79] A large number of interventions (n = 10)[17–21,26,32–34,36,40,42,48] did not target any one particular mental health diagnosis but instead covered general principles of diagnosis and treatment of child mental health concerns or involved embedding learners in clinics together such that they would see any range of mental health concerns that presented; all of these interventions are reported together as covering *general child mental health* in **Table 2**.

Included studies involved a relatively balanced mix of qualitative (n = 9),[26,28,31,33,35,37,40–42] quantitative (n = 8),[17,22,24,27,02,34,36,48] and mixed methods (n = 15)[18–21,23,25,29,30,38,39,43–47] designs. The most common modes of data collection were surveys (n = 20)[17,19–23,25–27,30,34,36–39,43,45–48] and/or interviews/focus groups (n = 14).[18,19,21,23,29–31,33,35,40,41,44,46,47] A minority of studies also employed observations or field notes of learners (n = 4)[19,21,29,31] or practice metrics such as clinic appointments, access to care, or billing data (n = 3).[18,24,32] Of the studies that used surveys, 13 developed their own forms,[17–19,21,26,27,34,36–39,45,46] and nine used or adapted previously published surveys, most commonly the Readiness for Interprofessional Learning Scale (n = 3).[22,25,39]

Educational Outcomes

Overall educational outcomes were skewed toward lower levels of outcomes on Kirkpatrick's pyramid (**Table 3**). Only seven studies reported patient- or systems-level outcomes (Level 4),[18,19,24,27,28,32,44] all of which were positive. Most notably, Pereira and colleagues[24] demonstrated a 91% decrease in emergency room visits for acute mental health crises after embedding psychology residents in a pediatric resident continuity clinic. Other studies reporting Level 4 outcomes were based on participant self-reports of improved patient treatment outcomes and referral networks being established[19,28]; practice-based metrics on the number of patients seen or treatments conducted in integrated care,[18,32] inpatient,[27] or dental[44] settings (without comparison metrics for what occurred prior to the IPE intervention); or other organizational outcome measures that could not be definitively attributed to the intervention described, such as clinic scholarly output[32] or the percentage of trainees who entered an interprofessional practice after graduation without a preintervention comparison.[18,32]

Eight studies[17–19,28,31,34,38,39] reported Level 3 outcomes. Of these, 6 were based on participants' self-report of behavior change after participation in IPE,[17,19,28,34,38,39] and two[18,31] were derived from other measures, specifically observations of trainee performance in an autism case simulation with standardized patients[31] and chart reviews and observations of pediatric trainees increasing rates of

Table 3
Intervention outcomes

Kirkpatrick Level	Total	Positive	Neutral/Mixed	Negative
Level 1: Reaction	16	13	3	0
Level 2: Knowledge, Skills, Attitudes	26	22	4	0
Level 3: Behavioral Change (Total)	8	8	0	0
Self-report only	6	6	0	0
Additional measure	2	2	0	0
Level 4: Patient- or Systems-level Outcome (Total)	7	7	0	0
Self-report only	2	2	0	0
Additional measure	5	5	0	0

referrals to and collaboration with psychologists within a resident continuity clinic.[18] No studies reported negative behavioral outcomes as a result of IPE.

The majority of studies reported Level 2 (n = 26)[17–20,22,23,25–27,29–31,33,34,36–39,41–48] or Level 1 (n = 16)[19–21,23,25,26,30,33,35,39–42,45–47] outcomes only. Studies reporting learner perceptions/reactions (Level 1) were positive overall, although a minority (n = 3)[30,35,40] reported learner critiques of some aspects of the training. Among studies assessing learner knowledge, attitudes, and skills (Level 2), all reported improvements related to the IPE intervention. However, four studies also reported minor negative or neutral findings, including a decrease[36] or no change[43] in knowledge scores, no changes in attitudes toward people with disabilities,[47] and unchanged attitudes toward IPE,[25] which the authors attributed to a ceiling effect as preintervention perceptions of IPE were already high.

DISCUSSION

This scoping review of IPE within CAMH describes the diversity of interventions—with respect to both the structure and content of the education delivered—that have been studied within this field. Across a range of clinical, school-based, and community-based settings and a variety of educational methods, CAMH IPE interventions were well received by participants and had overwhelmingly positive reported effects on learner attitudes, knowledge, and behaviors tied to IPE and interprofessional practice. However, this review also demonstrates that the majority of studies reported only lower-level educational outcomes, and it highlights important gaps that remain in our understanding of how best to implement CAMH IPE.

Importantly, a substantial number of interventions included not only medical and mental health professionals from a range of specialties but also a large number of allied health providers such as speech and occupational therapists and a broad range of nonhealthcare workers, including teachers, community youth workers, law enforcement, and even clergy. Accordingly, key findings from almost every study included some mention of improved understanding of other disciplines, role clarity, and/or professional collaboration, including expansion of referral networks and awareness of community resources. An estimated 20% of children experience significant mental health concerns, although only a small minority of those receive appropriate diagnosis and treatment in a medical setting.[9] Therefore, continuing to include diverse groups of participants in CAMH IPE from medical, educational, and community settings has the potential not only to enhance the training of participants immediately involved but also to expand the reach of professionals in multiple venues to help identify, support, and treat children with unmet mental health needs.

However, the breadth of CAMH topics addressed in IPE to date appears less robust. The vast majority covered either autism (n = 11)[22–25,28,29,31,43–46] or a range of general child mental health concerns without one specific focus (n = 10),[17–21,26,32–34,36,40,42,48] with far fewer covering anxiety (n = 5),[19–21,27,30,32,35] depression (n = 5),[19–21,24,30,32,35] or ADHD (n = 2),[24,32] for example, Yet this distribution is not reflective of the mental health diagnoses seen most frequently in pediatric primary care practice, in which ADHD, anxiety, and depression are seen much more frequently.[49] While the reasons for this incongruence are not clear, it is possible that the larger number of studies of IPE in autism is due to the greater likelihood of interdisciplinary team involvement in autism treatment as compared to ADHD, anxiety, or depression. Therefore, targeting future IPE interventions on some of these diagnoses that are more often encountered in general practice is an important area for future curriculum development and research.

Similar to findings from several other recently published literature reviews on IPE within mental health,[6,10–12] as well a more comprehensive review of IPE within medical education,[14] this current study found a preponderance of studies focusing on only learner reactions and attitudes as outcome measures. In addition, in accordance with these previous reviews, such lower-level learner outcomes were nearly all positive. It seems that participation in IPE—in almost any setting and delivery method studied—improves learner perceptions of and attitudes toward IPE. This current review therefore builds upon the argument that future IPE interventions do not need to keep asking these questions alone. Learner feedback and perceptions can still be valuable in future studies of IPE, but we would advocate that such outcomes should target more granular questions that are not so clearly answered by the current literature, such as, Which aspects of didactic IPE interventions are most high-yield, and why? In what circumstances are short-term IPE experiences valuable compared with when long-term or longitudinal engagement is needed? How can knowledge and attitude gains from short-term (nonlongitudinal) IPE interventions be sustained over time?

Yet if the ultimate goal of IPE is to improve learner readiness and competence for interprofessional practice in order to improve patient care, IPE interventions should strive toward patient- and systems-level outcomes that reflect this goal. Interestingly, except for one study involving simulation (31), all studies within this review that reported Level 3 or 4 outcomes, not based only on self-report, involved practice-based interventions (18, 24, 44, 27, 32). While for some types of participants in CAMH IPE (eg, nonmedical workers such as teachers or law enforcement), designing practice-based interventions with medical staff might be challenging or even impractical, community- and school-based partnerships could similarly provide venues for more practice-based interventions. Not only do practice-based interventions provide natural laboratories in which to measure patient- or organizational-level outcomes, but they also hold the potential to harness additional benefits to learning and identity formation. The theory of situated cognition suggests that learning is "situated" within a particular social and environmental context and cannot be separated from this context.[50] Specifically, Lave and Wenger[51] describe *communities of practice* in which learners (eg, medical residents or social work students) begin as more peripheral participants within a particular community (eg, a continuity clinic) and over time assume more central roles and responsibilities within it as they assimilate its attitudes, knowledge, and culture. Therefore, these theories would suggest that effective IPE must involve a degree of interprofessional practice in authentic practice environments in order to promote learning and to help instill in learners practice patterns and attitudes congruent with interprofessional practice.

This study has several limitations. First, as this paper was scoping review, although we did examine reported outcomes through the lens of Kirkpatrick's pyramid, we did not assess the papers themselves for quality, risk of bias, or levels of evidence. While these questions could be answered through a systematic review, it does not appear that the current state of the evidence for CAMH IPE is adequately established to support a systematic review. Second, many of the Level 3 or 4 outcomes reported were based on participant self-report and/or lacked preintervention comparisons. Therefore, while several papers reported behavioral, patient-level, or systems-level outcomes, in most cases it is not possible to definitely attribute these outcomes to the IPE intervention. Third, we only included English-language studies, so we could have missed findings from other regions globally. Finally, most papers included lacked a clear theoretic framework, so we were unable to meaningfully explore which educational theories have been helpful in guiding IPE interventions in CAMH to date. We hope this study can inspire and inform future IPE interventions in CAMH to expand the breadth of learners and topics involved and to strengthen future study designs.

SUMMARY

This scoping literature review identified 32 articles describing 29 IPE interventions in CAMH. Faculty or student/trainee physicians, psychologists, nurses, and social workers were the most common participants in IPE interventions, and physicians and psychologists the most frequent teachers, but many interventions also included a wide range of other mental health, allied health, educational, and community-based participants and teachers. Most interventions focused on autism or general child mental health and involved didactic and/or practice-based educational methods, with smaller numbers using observation or simulation. Outcomes reported from interventions revealed almost uniformly positive perceptions of training and attitudes toward IPE. A minority of studies did include higher-level outcomes such as behavioral changes or patient- or systems-level outcomes, although many of these outcomes were based on self-report and/or did not have preintervention comparisons. Future interventions in CAMH IPE should seek higher-level outcomes and strongly consider practice-based educational methods.

CLINICS CARE POINTS

- In designing interprofessional education (IPE) interventions in child and adolescent mental health (CAMH), educators can consider including a broad range of learner participants, including from allied health (eg, speech or occupational therapy) and nonmedical professions (eg, educators, community youth workers).

- More curriculum development and studies are needed on IPE interventions covering commonly seen pediatric mental health topics such as anxiety, depression, and ADHD.

- Interactive learning methods during didactic IPE sessions and practice-based IPE interventions are highly valued by participants.

- In accordance with theories of situated cognition, effective IPE is supported by authentic practice environments in which learners can assimilate practice patterns and attitudes congruent with interprofessional practice.

- Future studies of IPE should seek higher-level educational outcomes such as behavioral, patient-level, or systems-level changes, which might be easier to study and achieve using practice-based interventions.

DISCLAIMER

The views expressed in this article are those of the authors alone and do not represent the views of the United States Air Force, Department of Defense, or United States government.

DISCLOSURE

The authors have nothing to disclose.

SUPPLEMENTARY DATA

Supplementary data related to this article can be found online at https://doi.org/10.1016/j.chc.2021.07.001.

REFERENCES

1. Reeves S, Freeth D. Re-examining the evaluation of interprofessional education for community mental health teams with a different lens: understanding presage, process, and product factors. J Psychiatr Ment Health Nurs 2006;13(6):765–70.
2. Pauze E, Reeves S. Examining the effects of interprofessional education on mental health providers: findings from an updated systematic review. J Ment Health 2010;19(3):258–71.
3. Horwitz SM, Storfer-Isser A, Kerker BD, et al. Barriers to the identification and management of psychosocial problems: changes from 2004 to 2013. Acad Pediatr 2015;15(6):613–20.
4. Olson AL, Kelleher KJ, Kemper KJ, et al. Primary care pediatricians' roles and perceived responsibilities in the identification and management of depression in children and adolescents. Ambul Pediatr 2001;1:91–8.
5. Stein RE, Horwitz SM, Storfer-Isser A, et al. Do pediatricians think they are responsible for identification and management of child mental health problems? Results of the AAP periodic survey. Ambul Pediatr 2008;8:11–7.
6. Marcussen M, Norgaard B, Arnfred S. The effects of interprofessional education in mental health practice: findings from a systematic review. Acad Psych 2019; 43:200–8.
7. World Health Organization. Framework for action on interprofessional education & collaborative practice. Practice 2010;1–63. Available at: http://www.who.int/hrh/resources/framework_action/en/. Accessed February 21, 2021.
8. Martini R, Hilt R, Marx L, et al. Best principles for integration of child psychiatry into the pediatric health home 2012. Available at: https://www.aacap.org/App_Themes/AACAP/docs/clinical_practice_center/systems_of_care/best_principles_for_integration_of_child_psychiatry_into_the_pediatric_health_home_2012.pdf. Accessed 21 Febraury 2021.
9. American Academy of Child and Adolescent Psychiatry Committee on Health Care Access and Economics Task Force on Mental Health. Improving mental health services in primary care: reducing administrative and financial barriers to access and collaboration. Pediatr 2009;123(4):1248–51.
10. Landoll R, Maggio LA, Cervero RM, et al. Training the doctors: a scoping review of interprofessional education in primary care behavioral health (PCBH). J Clin Psychol Med Settings 2019;26:243–58.
11. Muzyk A, Smothers ZPW, Andolsek KM, et al. Interprofessional substance use disorder education in health professions education programs: a scoping review. Acad Med 2020;95(3):470–80.

12. Jackson M, Pelone F, Reeves S. Interprofessional education in the care of people diagnosed with dementia and their carers: a systematic review. BMJ Open 2016; 6(8):e010948.

13. Arksey H, O'Malley L. Scoping studies: towards a methodological framework. Int J Soc Res Methodol 2005;8:19–32.

14. Reeves S, Fletcher S, Barr H, et al. A BEME systematic review of the effects of interprofessional education: BEME guide no. 39. Med Teach 2016;38(7):656–68.

15. Kirkpatrick DL. Evaluating training programs: the four levels. San Francisco: Berrett-Koehler; 1994.

16. Levac D, Colquhoun H, O'Brien KK. Scoping studies: advancing the methodology. Implement Sci 2010;5:69.

17. Garfunkel LC, Pisani AR, leRoux P, et al. Educating residents in behavioral health care and collaboration: comparison of conventional and integrated training models. Acad Med 2011;86(2):174–9.

18. Pisani AR, LeRoux P, Siegel D. Educating residents in behavioral health care and collaboration: integrated clinical training of pediatric residents and psychology fellows. Acad Med 2011;86:166–73.

19. Church EA, Heath OJ, Curran VR, et al. Rural professionals' perceptions of interprofessional continuing education in mental health. Health Soc Care Community 2010;18(4):433–43.

20. Heath O, Church E, Curran V, et al. Interprofessional mental health training in rural primary care: findings from a mixed methods study. J Interprof Care 2015;29(3): 195–201.

21. Health OJ, Cornish PA, Callanan T, et al. Building interprofessional primary care capacity in mental health services in rural communities in Newfoundland and Labrador: an innovative training model. Can J Commun Ment Health 2008; 27(2):165–78.

22. Tsilimingras D, Gibson Scipio W, Clancy K, et al. Inteprofessional education during an autism session. J Commun Disord 2018;76:71–8.

23. Loutzenhiser L, Hadjistavropoulos H. Enhancing interprofessional patient-centered practice for children with autism spectrum disorders: a pilot project with pre-licensure health students. J Interprof Care 2008;22(4):429–31.

24. Pereira LM, Wallace J, Brown W, et al. Utilization and emergency department diversion as a result of pediatric psychology trainees integrated in pediatric primary and specialty clinics. Clin Pract Pediatr Psychol 2020.

25. Self TL, Parham DF. Students' self-perceptions of interprofessional education following participation on a diagnostic team for autism spectrum disorder. J Interprof Care 2016;30(5):682–4.

26. Splett J, Williams S, Reflections CL, et al. Learning by teaching: reflections on developing a curriculum for school mental health collaboration. Adv Sch Ment Health Promot 2011;4(2):27–38.

27. Gallagher KAS, McKenna K, Ibeziako P. Feasibility and impact of multidisciplinary training of an evidence-based intervention within a pediatric psychiatry consultation service. Acad Psychiatry 2014;38:445–50.

28. Clancy KM, Lipshultz SE. Training pediatric cardiologists to meet the needs of patients with neurodevelopmental disorders. Prog Pediatr Cardiol 2017;44:63–6.

29. Howell DM, Wittman P, Bundy MB. Interprofessional clinical education for occupational therapy and psychology students: a social skills training program for children with autism spectrum disorders. J Interprof Care 2012;26:49–55.

30. Iachini AL, Warren ME, Splett JW, et al. Exploring the impact of a pre-service interprofessional educational intervention for school mental health trainees. J Interprof Care 2015;29(2):162–4.
31. Kawamura A, Mylopoulos M, Orsino A, et al. Promoting the development of adaptive expertise: exploring a simulation model for sharing a diagnosis of autism with parents. Acad Med 2016;91:1576–81.
32. Kelsay K, Bunik M, Buchholz M, et al. Incorporating trainees' development into a multidisciplinary training model for integrated behavioral health within a pediatric continuity clinic. Child Adolesc Psychiatr Clin N Am 2017;26:703–15.
33. Priddis LE, Wells G. Innovations in interprofessional education and collaboration in a West Australian community health organisation. J Interprof Care 2011;25: 154–5.
34. Blanco-Vieria T, Silva Ribeiro W, Lauridsen-Ribeiro E, et al. An evaluation of a collaborative course for child and adolescent mental health professionals. J Interprof Care 2017;31(5):664–6.
35. Naismith LM, Kowalski C, Soklaridis S, et al. Participant perspectives on the contributions of physical, psychological, and sociological fidelity to learning in interprofessional mental health simulation. Simul Healthc 2020;15:141–6.
36. Carpenter J, Patsios D, Szilassy E, et al. Outcomes of short course interprofessional education in parental mental illness and child protection: self-efficacy, attitudes and knowledge. Soc Work Educ 2011;39(2):195–206.
37. Pettersen G, Rosenvinge JH, Thune-Larsen KB, et al. Clinical confidence following an interprofessional educational program on eating disorders for health care professionals: a qualitative analysis. J Multidiscip Healthc 2012;5:201–5.
38. Heath O, English D, Simms J, et al. Improving collaborative care in managing eating disorders. J Contin Educ Health Prof 2013;33(4):235–43.
39. McDevitt S, Passi V. Evaluation of a pilot interprofessional education programme for eating disorder training in mental health service. Ir J Psychol Med 2015;35: 289–99.
40. Vostanis P, O'Reilly M, Taylor H, et al. What can education teach child mental health services? Practitioners' perceptions of training and joint working. Emotional Behav Difficulties 2012;17:109–24.
41. Vostanis P, O'Reilly M, Duncan C, et al. Interprofessional training on resilience-building for children who experience trauma: Stakeholders' views from six low- and middle-income countries. J Interprof Care 2019;33(2):143–52.
42. Hegde S, Gajre MP, Shah H, et al. Interprofessional education and practice in an Indian setting. J Taibah Univ Med Sci 2017;12(3):265–7.
43. Beverly B, Wooster D. An interprofessional education initiative for allied health students preparing to serve individuals with autism spectrum disorders. J Allied Health 2018;47(2):90–5.
44. Anderson KL, Self TL, Carlson BN. Interprofessional collaboration of dental hygiene and communication sciences & disorders students to meet oral health needs of children with autism. J Allied Health 2017;46(4):e97–101.
45. Lewis A, Rudd CJ, Mills B. Working with children with autism: an interprofessional simulation-based tutorial for speech pathology and occupational therapy students. J Interprof Care 2018;32(2):242–4.
46. Brown LS, Benigno JP, Geist K. Come together: music therapy and speech-language pathology students' perspectives on collaboration during an inclusive camp for children with ASD. Music Ther Perspect 2018;36:17–25.
47. Iacono T, Lewis B, Tracy J, et al. DVD-based stories of people with developmental disabilities. Disabil Rehabil 2011;33(12):1010–21.

48. Acquavita SP, Lee BR, Levy M, et al. Preparing master of social work students for interprofessional practice. J Evid Based Soc Work 2020;17(5):611–23.
49. Mayne SL, Ross ME, Song L, et al. Variations in mental health diagnosis and prescribing across pediatric primary care pediatrics. Pediatr 2016;137(5): e20152974.
50. Durning SJ, Artino AR. Situativity theory: a perspective on how participants and the environment can interact: AMEE Guide no. 52. Med Teach 2011;33(3): 188–99.
51. Lave J, Wenger E. Situated learning: legitimate peripheral participation. Cambridge University Press; 1991.

The Role of the Child and Adolescent Psychiatrist in Systems of Care

Michael Sierra, MD*, Kaye McGinty, MD

KEYWORDS

• Child • Psychiatry • Role • System • Consultant

KEY POINTS

- Define "systems of care" as it pertains to child and adolescent psychiatry.
- Become familiar with the child-serving systems that make up the overarching system of care.
- Learn about the roles that child and adolescent psychiatry may have within and across systems of care.
- Become a catalyst for system improvement.

INTRODUCTION

To adequately answer the question, "what is the role of the child and adolescent psychiatrist (CAP) in systems of care?," one would first have to answer multiple implicit questions. What is a system or system of care? What are the child-serving systems that make up the system of care? What are the roles a CAP could have within and across these systems? How might the CAP's role change to adapt to current or anticipated challenges? This article aims to answer these implicit questions and provide a satisfactory answer for the original question.

DISCUSSION
What Is a System or System of Care?

A system is defined as "a collection of interdependent elements that interact to achieve a common purpose."[1] As it pertains to child and adolescent psychiatry, a system of care is "a spectrum of effective, community-based services and supports for children and youths with or at risk for mental health or other challenges and their families, that is organized into a coordinated network, builds meaningful partnerships with

Division of Child and Adolescent Psychiatry, Department of Psychiatry, Prisma Health, Greenville, SC 29605, USA
* Correspondence.
E-mail address: Michael.Sierra@primsahealth.org

Child Adolesc Psychiatric Clin N Am 30 (2021) 727–736
https://doi.org/10.1016/j.chc.2021.06.002
1056-4993/21/© 2021 Elsevier Inc. All rights reserved.

families and youth, and addresses their cultural and linguistic needs, in order to help them to function better at home, in school, in the community, and throughout life."[2] With this understanding, a CAP may begin to adopt "systems thinking," which is a style of thinking and problem-solving that empowers a clinician to adopt a broad-based understanding of clinical concerns, recognize the properties of the system or systems involved in patient care, and make more meaningful connections within and across systems.[3] When devising a treatment plan, the psychiatrist who possesses systems thinking will go beyond recommending psychopharmacologic and psycho-therapeutic interventions and also consider the systems involved in supporting the youth and family, interface with these systems effectively, and work to improve the functioning within and across these systems.

What Are the Child-Serving Systems that Make up the System of Care?

There are 8 child-serving systems relevant to the CAP: the education system, primary health care system, public mental health system, child welfare system, juvenile justice system, developmental disabilities system, substance abuse treatment services system, and early childhood services system.[3] This section provides an introduction to these systems and discusses how their current structure may influence the role of a CAP.

The Education System

Approximately 60% of all youths who received mental health services during their lives entered via the education system.[4] About 8% of adolescents meet criteria for a serious emotional disturbance, yet only one-third to one-half of children and adolescents with emotional and behavioral disorders receive mental health services.[5] Therefore, the education system has the potential to play a pivotal role in reducing gaps in treatment access. As such, many CAPs work in schools either as clinicians or as consultants. These roles allow the CAP to work with school teams to create school programs that promote mental health and resiliency, decrease barriers to access and stigma, and increase opportunities for early intervention, treatment, and prevention.[6]

The Primary Care System

Primary care, which includes a variety of outpatient, inpatient, and in-home health care settings, plays an important role in identifying, treating, and referring children with mental health problems. Because of the shortage of CAPs, stigma surrounding mental health, and barriers that may prevent a patient from following through with a referral to mental health, primary care providers (PCPs) have assumed the care of many youths with mental health disorders and have become partners with CAPs. To address these issues, some CAPs are using a different service delivery model by integrating mental health services with primary care services. Examples of integrative models include colocated models, where the CAP works within the primary care office. The University of Washington's Advanced Integrated Mental Health Solutions Center developed Collaborative Care, a specific type of integrated care model, where patients with persistent mental illness who require systematic follow-up are placed in a registry, tracked using measurement-based practice, and treated to a target. Trained PCPs and other professionals provide evidence-based biopsychosocial treatments and are supported by regular psychiatric case consultations for patients who are not improving as expected. This model has been shown to improve patient outcomes, improve patient satisfaction, and reduce cost.[7]

The Public Mental Health System

The community mental health services within the public mental health system play an important role in addressing the mental health needs of communities. The overall mission of this system is to address the morbidity and mortality caused by mental illness. For children and adolescents, special attention is given to those with severely impairing and chronic conditions, those with limited access to care, and those involved with other public sector systems like child welfare or juvenile justice. Youths with developmental disabilities or substance abuse are excluded from the target population of the public mental health system if these disorders occur in isolation but may be served by the public mental health system if they have a cooccurring disorder that requires mental health interventions. The array of services provided by the public mental health system typically spans a continuum of care. A traditional care continuum would include prevention and early intervention programs, consultations with schools and other agencies, office-based clinical services, day treatment programs, partial hospitalization, residential services (both short term and long term), acute hospitalization and crisis intervention services, and long-term state hospitalization services. More robust systems will have additional elements, including wraparound teams, paraprofessional services, intensive case management, and care coordination. Interventions included in the wraparound plan of care are most likely to be effective when the treatment services are evidence-based and provided by skilled clinicians. There is an emphasis on strengths-based care that highlights, identifies, and builds on the competence of youth and their families during all phases of treatment. A broad continuum of care helps provide services needed to augment natural supports of youth and families and improve the youth's functioning at home, in school, and in the community. The CAP's role within the public mental health system is broad, including diagnostic assessment, treatment, and team-based services. With the development of the continuum of care, it is helpful for the CAP to also serve on wraparound and in-home treatment teams, as well as consulting to care management organizations that provide some of the care.

The Child Welfare System

The child welfare system is made up of "a continuum of services designed to protect children, strengthen families to care for their children, and promote permanency when children cannot remain with or return to their families."[8] Up to 80% of youths served by the child welfare system, particularly those in foster care, have a mental or behavioral health problem requiring intervention.[9] A CAP often interfaces with this system while fulfilling the role of a mandated reporter in cases of suspected child maltreatment. Trauma and adverse childhood experiences can have effects on a child's neurobiology, psychosocial development, and functioning.[10,11] When caring for youths being served by the child welfare system, the CAP should be aware of the youth's legal status and who has the authority to consent for evaluation and treatment. CAPs treat many youths in state custody in the typical clinical settings, but also are consultants at child welfare group homes and residential facilities and serve on child welfare wraparound teams.

The Juvenile Justice System

The juvenile justice system aims to simultaneously protect public safety and hold justice-involved youths accountable for their actions, while providing services to the youth and family that would help youths live productive and law-abiding lives. Youths can enter the juvenile justice system for criminal offenses or status offenses. Status offenses are noncriminal acts that violate the law only because the person committing them is a minor (ie, truancy). Status offending may be a sign of underlying psychosocial risk factors that put the youth at greater risk of further delinquency, physical health issues, mental health issues, and addiction.[12] Within the juvenile justice system, the CAP may be recruited for the role of expert witness or forensic evaluator. An expert witness is often asked to perform a forensic evaluation as specified by the court, and to share their opinion based on their findings with the court. These evaluations are not part of the therapeutic process, and a CAP should never have the dual role of treating clinician and forensic evaluator because of the inherent conflict of interest. CAPs may treat youths in this system in outpatient settings, as these youths are kept at home, or as consultants in juvenile justice group homes, residential treatment centers, or secure custody facilities.

The Substance Abuse Treatment Services System

The substance abuse treatment services system is also an important child-serving system. More than 20% of eighth graders have abused a substance in their lifetime, and more than 20% of 12 graders have used a substance within the last month.[13] Adolescent substance abuse is associated with sexually risky behavior, trauma, mental health disorders, and suicide.[14] Despite the prevalence of substance abuse disorders (SUDs) cooccurring with mental health disorders, organizational and fiscal factors on a state and local level often fracture substance abuse services from mental health services. This fracture often makes individuals with SUDs and cooccurring psychiatric illness misfits within the systems of care because regulatory, licensing, and reimbursement barriers impede successful integration between substance abuse and mental health services.[15] There are many opportunities for CAPs to work with this population in outpatient substance abuse services settings and residential treatment programs.

The Developmental Disabilities Service System

Developmental disabilities services pose challenges because, throughout the United States, there are many different configurations of state-sponsored services and significant variability in eligibility requirements.[16] This variability can create barriers for children with intellectual disability and autism, especially if the family is moving to a new state or region. The CAP must have a good understanding of the organizational structure and eligibility requirements of these services on a state and local level, and use case managers when possible to help caregivers connect youths with developmental disabilities to appropriate services. When serving a youth with a developmental disability, transitioning from child services to adult services is critically important. A youth with a developmental disability may need permanent guardianship. The CAP should be willing and able to assess the youth's decision-making ability and guardianship needs at the transition point. Furthermore, CAPs have opportunities within this system to provide outpatient care, collaborate with developmental-behavioral pediatrics and family teams, and provide consultations at group homes and residential treatment facilities.

The Early Childhood Services System

Much like the developmental disabilities services system, the early childhood system is a difficult one to navigate because of its complex service array that varies from state to state. This system tends to include early intervention services, which focus on creating individualized and multidisciplinary treatment plans to improve the functioning of young children (ages 0–3 years) with intellectual disability, genetic conditions, syndromes, cerebral palsy, or those who are at risk of developing developmental disabilities, and special education services, which assist children ages 3 to 21 whose disability interferes with their ability to benefit from general classroom instruction.[17] The early childhood system has opportunities for the CAP to perform consultations at childcare facilities and developmental centers, and be a member of child and family teams.

What Are the Roles a Child and Adolescent Psychiatrist Could Have Within and Across These Systems?

As many CAPs understand, the child-serving systems are serving many youths who are in dire need of child psychiatric clinical services. As such, most CAPs that are working in systems act as clinical providers who evaluate, diagnose, and treat patients; this can include prescribing psychopharmacologic treatments, performing psychotherapy, and helping the child and family connect with appropriate services via referrals or system navigation. Clinical providers should be familiar with their local child-serving systems and adopt the Child and Adolescent Social Service Program Core principles of providing youth-guided, family-focused, community-based, multisystem, culturally competent, and least-restrictive care. These principles have provided an organizing framework for the public mental health system for more than 20 years.[18] Assessing for and cultivating the strengths of the youth and family as well as helping them develop their networks of natural supports is an essential system of care focus. As a system, it is essential to change the conversation from sickness and disability to strengths, wellness, and resiliency. This mindset helps the youth, families, and system partners find renewed energy and consider new strategies. The CAP is essential in promoting this mindset and helping guide the team members as they develop these skills. This is just the beginning of the CAP role.

The CAP working in systems will often have the role of a teacher. A CAP may be recruited to educate others regarding their areas of expertise. Their most important role is learning from and helping the youth and family understand the diagnostic impressions, treatment recommendations, and the systems they are navigating. Learners may include students from many different disciplines, and it is vital for them to see how the CAP works within the system. System employees can also benefit from the CAP's expertise. Many of the child-serving systems use interdisciplinary or multidisciplinary teams, which provide brief educational opportunities. At other times, the CAP may be asked to do formal trainings or recruit others with expertise in certain areas. The system administrators may also ask the CAP regarding their knowledge about outside training, and the CAP should provide their most educated response. A CAP will simultaneously be an active listener and learner and should work to gather systems knowledge about people, programs, and populations pertinent to the system or systems with which they interface.

As the CAP continues to work with system partners in collaboration with youth and families, advocacy on many different levels is important. A CAP should never assume someone else is advocating. Most CAPs are accustomed to advocating for individual youth and/or family level needs, and this may occur in any system. Once the CAP works with a specific system for some time, they may find opportunities to advocate for programs, funding, and other system issues, which are impacting the delivery of care to the youth and family. The CAP may be on local/state committees or task forces and may have opportunities to use those forums for advocacy. Other times, advocacy may occur at the legislative or policy level. The CAP will usually require additional learning and allies from different professions to effectively engage in this type of advocacy. The 2 most important advocacy roles for the CAP regarding working in systems is having the gravitas to speak up for the youth and families when no one else can or will, and to be looking for opportunities for system change and improvements when everyone else is working on the details of the system mission. An important advocacy point that has become more apparent is youths involved in child-serving systems have a disproportionately high rate of trauma exposure and greater impairments at baseline compared with other youths.[19,20] When trauma goes unrecognized, the interventions may be less effective. Trauma-informed care is a public health concept that involves a specific set of beliefs about individuals, organizations, and systems, and a related set of practices, all intended to prevent and mitigate the impact of trauma.[21] CAPs need to advocate for trauma-informed care in all child-serving systems.

As CAPs progress in their careers, many realize that their impact can only go so far at the individual and family level. They begin desiring to impact the broader population and get involved at a more global level. This type of work can lead to enormous professional satisfaction and improve a system's response to the needs of youth and families with mental health challenges. Therefore, it is important for the CAP to consider, strategize, and seek mentorship to develop as a system consultant over time. System leaders understand that an experienced CAP's contributions and creativity will help develop solutions that will better meet the needs of those served by the system and overcome system challenges. To be an effective consultant to the system, a CAP must be knowledgeable about the system mandates, procedures, requirements, funding, external barriers, and internal challenges. Through this process, the CAP will become a valuable team member who can form relationships and become a resource for important individuals within the system. These relationships develop over time and should be thought of as a long-term process. As a system-level team member, the CAP provides important expertise while learning as much from the other team members. In this role, the CAP may be asked to provide an administrative-based consultation. Administrative-based consultations do not center on a patient, but rather on an organization or agency. Administrative-based consultations may help organizations in various ways. Some examples include joining a team involved in program development and evaluation, guiding systematic changes to improve the effectiveness of existing programs, evaluating the effectiveness of staff in achieving goals regarding the target population of youths, and participating in development or selection of prevention strategies to use with the youth in care. An important role of a consultant is also that of a liaison. Although the distinction between the role of a liaison and a consultant is not always clear, a liaison develops an ongoing relationship with the consultee and/or youth and family. A liaison works to enhance the communication, cooperation, and cohesion of a team through teaching and interpersonal effectiveness. The role of a liaison may help reduce the distress of team members, youth, and families and improve the systematic response toward youths with mental health problems.

Although many CAPs will remain as consultants to child-serving systems of care, a few CAPs will be recruited to serve as administrators for local, state, and federal agencies who serve youth populations. These CAPs have usually had previous experience in child-serving systems and developed important relationships at the local or state level. These CAPs work closely with other administrators at the state level and have various roles regarding policy, practice guidelines, and regulatory measures. They also serve on many committees or task forces for legislatures or state government to address specific problems related to youth and families. CAP system administrators promote the use of a population health approach within child-serving services. As most CAPs realize, the systems of care need to promote prevention and wellness so that all system professionals will care for each youth and family in their charge as if they were their own family.

How Might the Child and Adolescent Psychiatrist's Roles Change to Adapt to Current and Anticipated Challenges?

Many of the child-serving systems face challenges when attempting to meet the needs of their communities. These challenges often stem from an insufficient work-force, limited resources, a lack of integration across systems, and a narrowed focus on treating illness and resolving crisis (without sufficient attention to population health, promotion of wellness, and community supports). In the United States, there is less than one-fourth of the CAPs needed to address the estimated national need.[22] In the past 2 decades, the number of emergency room visits for child psychiatric emergencies has nearly doubled as the national availability of pediatric inpatient psychiatric beds has fallen over that same time.[23,24] The high turnover of child welfare workers and wraparound care coordinators may undermine rehabilitation and treatment efforts.[25–27] Integrated models of care and interdisciplinary treatment planning face administrative and financial barriers, which fragments care.[28] As opposed to other medical specialties, preventative interventions in child and adolescent psychiatry are often viewed as diverting resources and finances away from individuals with active mental illness or thought to have minimal long-term impacts.[29] To make matters worse, the COVID-19 outbreak began December of 2019 and resulted in a global pandemic that, at the time of this writing, continues to negatively impact most countries. COVID-19 has led to unpredictability, uncertainty, social isolation, loss of income, inactivity, limited access to services, increased access to alcohol, and decreased social support, further increasing known risk factors for mental health problems, domestic violence, and child abuse and neglect.[30] Attempts to implement infection-control measures resulted in shutdowns of schools and other important service settings, created barriers to delivering services, increased the use of remote delivery models, and lead to an economic breakdown that impacted the available budget for many child-serving systems.

In response to these challenges, a CAP has the role of working to increase the mental health workforce globally and nationally. CAPs will need to make efforts to improve the desirability of pursuing a career in mental health and reduce stigma. To meet the growing mental health demands, the workforce will likely evolve into multidisciplinary services with teams that include CAPs, PCPs, other specialty physicians, social workers, psychologists, other professionals, and paraprofessionals. A CAP's service time will likely trend toward performing initial diagnostic assessments and consultations, caring for the youth with the most severe disorders, and supporting allied professionals and paraprofessionals who care for youths with mild to moderate mental health disorders. CAPs will need to continue to provide telehealth services when possible, to improve access to care for all youths. CAPs will need to adopt roles that research, demonstrate, and implement effective prevention and early interventions that have substantial long-term value, decrease the use of future intensive and more expensive services, and reduce the burden of child and adolescent psychiatric disorders. CAPs must become members of public health initiatives that promote system integration and interagency collaboration, population health, the healthy development of youths, and supportive parenting. For example, a CAP may partner with schools to implement mental health literacy programs that promote resilience in children and families, or join advocacy groups that support legislative action that would remove barriers that prevent the successful integration of mental health and substance abuse services. The CAP will have the important role of collaborating with system partners to advocate for and help the child-serving systems adjust to the challenges and economic breakdowns caused or exacerbated by the COVID-19 pandemic.

SUMMARY

A CAP's role in systems of care grows and evolves over time. It begins with understanding systems and systems of care, adopting systems thinking, and becoming familiar with state and local child-serving systems. Early career roles usually focus on providing clinical services and grow to include teaching, advocating, acquiring more systems knowledge, and discovering opportunities to become a systems consultant. The system of care must continue to treat youth and families with active mental health problems, but also adequately promote population health through effective early intervention and prevention programs that keep more youths in the home, at school, and in the community. The CAP will have a role in promoting this mindset through research, advocacy, interagency collaboration, and multidisciplinary planning. The child-serving systems face many financial and logistical barriers that hinder avenues of necessary growth, and many of these barriers have been exacerbated by the COVID-19 pandemic. The CAP will play an important role in collaborating with system partners to find solutions to overcome the many challenges and barriers present and to promote youth and family empowerment and wellness.

CLINICS CARE POINTS

- Child and adolescent psychiatrists are important contributors in child-serving systems of care and may have many roles.
- Child and adolescent psychiatrists serving as consultants to systems is growing in importance.
- Child and adolescent psychiatrist system consultants will promote a population health approach to include advocacy, early intervention and prevention programs, and youth and family empowerment and wellness.

DISCLOSURE

The authors have no disclosures nor conflict of interests.

REFERENCES

1. Nolan TW. Understanding medical systems. Ann Intern Med 1998;128:293–8.
2. Stroul B, Blau G, Friedman R. Updating the system of care concept and philosophy. Washington, DC: Georgetown University Center for Child and Human Development, National Technical Assistance Center for Children's Mental Health; 2010. Available at: http://www.socflorida.com/documents/professionals/06-17_updating_SOC_concept&philosophy.pdf. Accessed February 27, 2021.
3. American Academy of Child and Adolescent Psychiatry. Training toolkit for systems-based practice. Process modules. Systems-based practice overview. 2019. Available at: https://www.aacap.org/App_Themes/AACAP/docs/resources_for_primary_care/training_toolkit_for_systems_based_practice/Overview-Module-August-2019-(8.19.19).pdf. Accessed February 21, 2021.
4. Farmer EM, Burns BJ, Phillips SD, et al. Pathways into and through mental health services for children and adolescents. Psychiatr Serv 2003;54(1):60–6.

5. Green JG, Xuan Z, Kwong L, et al. School referral patterns among adolescents with serious emotional disturbance enrolled in systems of care. J Child Fam Stud 2016;25(1):290–8.
6. Stephan SH, Weist M, Kataoka S, et al. Transformation of children's mental health services: the role of school mental health. Psychiatr Serv 2007;58(10):1330–8.
7. Archer J, Bower P, Gilbody S, et al. Collaborative care for people with depression and anxiety. Cochrane Database Syst Rev 2012;(10).
8. Child welfare information gateway glossary. Available at: https://www.childwelfare.gov/glossary/glossaryc/. Accessed February 21, 2021.
9. Pecora PJ, Jensen PS, Hunter Romanelli L, et al. Mental health services for children placed in foster care: an overview of current challenges. Child Welfare 2009; 88:5–26.
10. Van de Kolk B. The neurobiology of childhood trauma and abuse. Child Adolesc Psychiatr Clin N Am 2003;121(2):293–317.
11. Centers for Disease Control and Prevention. Adverse childhood experiences study 2005.
12. Development Services Group, Inc.. "Status offenders." Literature review. Washington, DC: Office of Juvenile Justice and Delinquency Prevention; 2015. https://www.ojjdp.gov/mpg/litreviews/Status_Offenders.pdf. Accessed February 24, 2021.
13. National Institute on Drug Abuse. Monitoring the future study: Trends in prevalence of various drugs. 2020. Available at: https://www.drugabuse.gov/drug-topics/trends-statistics/monitoring-future/monitoring-future-study-trends-in-prevalence-various-drugs. Accessed February 27, 2021.
14. Centers for Disease Control and Prevention. Youth risk behavior survey: data summary & trends report 2009 – 2019. Available at: https://www.cdc.gov/healthyyouth/data/yrbs/pdf/YRBSDataSummaryTrendsReport2019-508.pdf. Accessed February 27, 2021.
15. Minkoff K, Cline C. Changing the world: the design and implementation of comprehensive continuous integrated systems of care for individuals with co-occurring disorders. Psychiatr Clin N Am 2004;27(4):727–43.
16. American Academy of Child and Adolescent Psychiatry. Training toolkit for systems-based practice. System modules. Developmental disabilities system. 2009. Available at: https://www.aacap.org/App_Themes/AACAP/docs/resources_for_primary_care/training_toolkit_for_systems_based_practice/p%20-%20Systems%20Based%20Practice%20Module%20-%20Developmental%20Disabilities%20For%20Web.pdf. Accessed February 27, 2021.
17. American Academy of Child and Adolescent Psychiatry. Training toolkit for systems-based practice. System modules. Early childhood services system. 2009. Available at: https://www.aacap.org/App_Themes/AACAP/docs/resources_for_primary_care/training_toolkit_for_systems_based_practice/r%20-%20Systems%20Based%20Practice%20Module%20-%20Early%20Childhood%20For%20Web.pdf. Accessed February 27, 2021.
18. Pennsylvania Department of Human Services. Child and adolescent social service program (CASSP). Available at: https://www.dhs.pa.gov/Services/Mental-Health-In-PA/Pages/CASSP.aspx. Accessed February 27, 2021.
19. Whitson ML, Connell CM. The relation of exposure to traumatic events and longitudinal mental health outcomes for children enrolled in systems of care: results from a national system of care evaluation. Am J Community Psychol 2016; 57(3–4):380–90.

20. Snyder FJ, Roberts YH, Crusto CA, et al. Exposure to traumatic events and the behavioral health of children enrolled in an early system of care. J Traumatic Stress 2012;25(6):700–4.
21. Substance Abuse and Mental Health Services Administration. SAMHSA's concept of trauma and guidance for a trauma-informed approach. Rockville MD: Substance Abuse Mental Health Services Administration; 2014.
22. American Academy of Child and Adolescent Psychiatry (AACAP). Child and adolescent psychiatry workforce crisis: solutions to improve early intervention and access to care. Washington, DC: AACAP; 2013. Available at: https://www.aacap.org/App_Themes/AACAP/docs/Advocacy/policy_resources/cap_workforce_crisis_201305.pdf. Accessed February 27, 2021.
23. Hazen EP, Prager LM. A quiet crisis: pediatric patients waiting for inpatient psychiatric care. J Am Acad Child Adolesc Psychiatry 2017;56:631–3.
24. Carubia B, Becker A, Levine BH. Child psychiatric emergencies: updates on trends, clinical care, and practice challenges. Curr Psychiatry Rep 2016; 18(4):41.
25. Brown. The central role of relationships with trauma-informed integrated care for children and youth. Acad Pediatr 2017;17(7):S94–101.
26. Strolin-Goltzman J, Kollar S, Trinkle J. Listening to the voices of children in foster care: youths speak out about child welfare workforce turnover and selection. Soc Work 2010;55(1):47–53.
27. Walker JS, Schurer Coldiron J, Taylor E. Turnover among wraparound care coordinators: stakeholders' views on causes, impacts, and remedies. The National Technical Assistance Network for Children's Behavioral Health;. Baltimore, MD: The; 2017.
28. National Technical Assistance Network for Children's Behavioral Health. Available at: https://nwi.pdx.edu/pdf/Turnover-Among-Wraparound-Care-Coordinators.pdf. Accessed February 27, 2021.
29. Stiffman AR, Stelk W, Horwitz SM, et al. A public health approach to children's mental health services: possible solutions to current service inadequacies. Adm Policy Ment Health 2010;37(1–2):120–4.
30. Moreno C, Wykes T, Galderisi S, et al. How mental health care should change as a consequence of the COVID-19 pandemic. Lancet Psychiatry 2020;7(9):813–24.

A Public Partnership to Support Well-Being

Population Health Implementation of Trauma and Resilience Informed Care Across Child and Family Ecosystems

Patricia Lester, MD[a], Catherine Mogil, PsyD[a],*,
Norweeta Milburn, PhD[a], Gita Murthy, MSW, MPH, LCSW[b],
Jonathan Sherin, MD, PhD[c]

KEYWORDS

- Child and family well-being • Equity • Implementation • Learning system
- Population health • Public mental health partnership • Resilience • Trauma-informed

KEY POINTS

- A public health response to build resilience and mitigate the impact of adversity and trauma in children and families requires a population-level approach across community ecosystems and service systems.
- Implementation science and participatory community approaches provide important insights to develop population-level trauma and resilience informed practices driven by a culture of continuous improvement.
- Partnerships between public community mental health and research universities working alongside communities and families are optimally positioned to advance well-being in children and families.
- University-community partnerships that create a culture of reciprocal learning honoring lived experience and practice-based evidence can advance equity and well-being in marginalized and underresourced communities.

[a] UCLA Department of Psychiatry and Biobehavioral Sciences, 760 Westwood Plaza, A8-159, Los Angeles, CA 90024, USA; [b] Los Angeles County Department of Mental Health + UCLA Strike Team, 3261 Lincoln Avenue, Altadena, CA 91001, USA; [c] Los Angeles County Department of Mental Health, 11301 Wilshire Boulevard, Los Angeles, CA 90073, USA
* Corresponding author.
E-mail address: CMogil@mednet.ucla.edu

Child Adolesc Psychiatric Clin N Am 30 (2021) 737–750
https://doi.org/10.1016/j.chc.2021.07.002
1056-4993/21/© 2021 Elsevier Inc. All rights reserved.

childpsych.theclinics.com

Abbreviations	
DMH	LA County Department of Mental Health
LA	Los Angeles
PPFW	DMH + UCLA Public Partnership for Wellbeing
Prevention COE	DMH + UCLA Prevention Center of Excellence
TRIC	trauma and resilience informed care
UCLA	University of California at Los Angeles

INTRODUCTION

Experiences of early life adversity and trauma are a threat to child, youth and family well-being. Consistent with decades of research documenting the cumulative risk of early childhood adversity,[1] the last two decades have documented that adverse childhood experiences are associated with negative health and mental health outcomes in adulthood, as well as lower educational and economic attainment.[2–4] Prior research has found that early life stressors (including child maltreatment such as physical and sexual abuse, and family dysfunction such as domestic violence, mental illness, and incarceration) are among the strongest known determinants of mental and physical well-being throughout life, particularly for children living in poverty.[2,5] Adverse experiences during development contribute to heightened neural sensitivity to threats that can promote dysregulation of the sympathetic nervous system, hypothalamic–pituitary–adrenal axis, and immune system and lead to increased inflammation and substantial disparities in lifelong individual risk for many disease conditions, including anxiety disorders, depression, heart disease, diabetes, cancer, and autoimmune and neurodegenerative disorders.[6,7] Additional traumatic experiences during childhood and adolescence, such as community violence, disasters, war, racism, and other emotionally harmful events also increase the risk of sequelae across a range of well-being outcomes.[8–11]

The need to both prevent and address early adversity and trauma is increasingly recognized as foundational to public health at a population level.[12] A comprehensive public health response to build individual, family, and community resilience and mitigate adversity and trauma requires a tiered, population-level approach that includes mental health promotion, prevention, screening, early intervention, and effective assessment and treatment across community ecosystems and services.[13] Creating a trauma-responsive community ecosystem includes developing knowledge, skills, and processes needed to implement the principles of trauma and resilience informed care (TRIC) as well as the time and support necessary to maintain them within organizational cultures, practices, and policies.[14,15] This process relies on building meaningful and sustainable partnerships that support collaboration among individuals, families, and providers at individual, organizational, and systems levels. Sustained and meaningful engagement of leadership, partners, staff, families, and youth is needed to address intersections of race, history, gender, and language as well as the compounding impact of systemic racism and inequities on diverse communities. Additionally, sustainable trauma-responsive systems necessitate maintaining an environment of support for the workforce in order to reduce secondary traumatic stress, burnout, and moral distress and promote staff resilience and well-being.[16] Decades of research on child development, preventive interventions, and trauma and adversity provide the foundational catalyst for developing a population-level framework to support well-being in children and families.[12,17–20]

The largest mental health agency in the United States—the Los Angeles (LA) County Department of Mental Health (DMH)—and the University of California at Los Angeles

(UCLA), both of which are large public-serving institutions, have partnered to advance the well-being of LA County by strengthening communities, reengineering service systems, and revitalizing mental health policy with a focus on racial equity. This manuscript provides an overview of a foundational population health approach to building trauma and resilience informed ecosystems to support child and family well-being through a continuum of mental health services. We describe the specific need and development of the LA County DMH + UCLA Public Partnership for Wellbeing (PPFW). Next, we provide a roadmap with core principles from this partnership and actionable steps that could be used to implement this approach for children, youth, and family well-being in other parts of the United States to integrate more coherent, comprehensive, and adaptive support systems into the community ecosystems where families live, work, learn, and play. We conclude with a summary of both lessons learned and opportunities to advance this approach leveraged by community and academic partnerships.

Role of Promotion, Prevention, and Continuum of Services That Are Culturally Humble and Trauma-Informed in Strengthening Communities

Mental health preventive interventions that promote resilience processes have been shown to reduce the burden of mental health problems for individuals, families, and communities at risk due to a range of adversity across development. A trauma and resilience informed approach to prevention involves strengthening protective factors, skills, and social connections while reducing risk factors and stressors.[21] Research demonstrates that prioritizing mental health promotion and prevention can mitigate negative long-term outcomes of adversity as well as promote well-being for children and their families.[22] A trauma-responsive system depends upon fostering shared responsibility for youth and families across service systems and ecosystems that support families within communities, and improving interagency communication and coordination, in part bolstered by resources for interdisciplinary training and implementation.

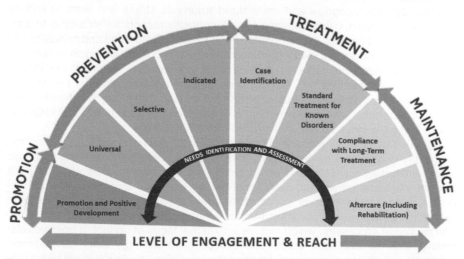

Fig. 1. A continuum of well-being support for children and families. National Academies of Sciences, Engineering, and Medicine. 2019. Strengthening the Military Family Readiness System for a Changing American Society. https://doi.org/10.17226/25380. (Reproduced with permission from the National Academy of Sciences, Courtesy of the National Academies Press, Washington, DC).

A population health framework for enhancing child and family well-being across community systems includes a continuum of support that promotes positive development, screening, prevention, and early intervention as well as timely treatment and recovery services. Prevention includes strategies to promote well-being as well as reduce the impact of trauma and adversity not only on the child but also across the caregiver and family system.[23] This continuum of prevention has been adapted from the Gordon 1983 model (ie, universal, selective, and indicated). This model has been incorporated into multiple national prevention reports[19,24] as a tiered continuum of mental health support (**Fig. 1**; adapted from the National Academies of Sciences, Engineering, and Medicine, 2016,[25] 2019[26]). The model includes a specific focus on engagement, measurement, and promotional activities that reinforce resilience processes within children and families within community ecosystems and service systems.

Implementation of a Trauma-Informed Prevention Framework

A trauma-informed prevention framework addresses the far-reaching impact of adverse and traumatic events on individuals, families, communities, and systems by increasing awareness and developing knowledge of practices that promote healing and recovery. As described by the Substance Abuse and Mental Health Services Administration,[27] trauma-informed care fosters safety, builds transparency and trustworthiness, encourages collaboration, leverages peer support, promotes voice and empowerment, and includes attention to cultural, historical, and gender issues. Adoption of a population-level trauma-informed framework requires integration of these principles into policies that shape children's and families' lives, as well as alignment of practices throughout the ecosystems that support them. The adoption of an entire service system to be trauma-informed indicates that all service providers are responsive to potential traumatic stress on people who are engaged in that system.[15] Although one cannot be sure who has experienced trauma, the goal is to treat all children, family members, caregivers, and other residents with the same care as if they had experienced a trauma.[28] It also indicates that agencies and organizations within a service system recognize and understand traumatic stress and work to reduce the burden of trauma, using evidence-based, culturally responsive strategies to support recovery and healing. Finally, systems that foster collaboration and mutuality can more effectively address the intersection of trauma and culture, historical racism and oppression, gender, and linguistic diversity to be responsive to the needs of children, families, and communities.[15,27] Workforce development training practices must similarly follow these principles so that all efforts are infused with safety, trustworthiness, mutual collaboration, and empowerment with attention given to cultural and historical factors that have played a role in the development of identity.

In addition to the healing power of trauma-informed practices, service systems and community ecosystems have an opportunity to adopt resilience-promoting practices to prevent further adversity and equip individuals and communities with the skills necessary to foster growth and overall well-being. Resilience is defined as the capacity of a system to rebound or successfully adapt following adverse experiences.[29] Research indicates some common themes among studies of individual and family level resilience processes, which include an internal locus of control, a positive relationship with at least one adult, effective problem-solving, social competence, perceived self-efficacy, emotionally responsive parenting, guiding cultural belief systems, and an ability to make positive meaning out of adversity.[29–32] While initially understood as individually-based, resilience research has been expanded to better understand diverse systems, including families, businesses, communities, and economies.[33] Magis (2010)[34] has defined community resilience as "the existence, development, and engagement of community resources by community members to thrive in an environment characterized by change, uncertainty, unpredictability, and surprise." Community resilience has a symbiotic relationship with the individuals within that community. In other words, a group of resilient individuals are likely to develop resilient communities, and resilient communities are likely to support the development of individual resilience.[13]

Resilience promotion relies on the availability and deployment of effective community resources, engagement of change agents for strategic collective action, equitable resource allocation, and positive impact.[34] Each community resource must also be trauma-informed and resilience-promoting within its own governance and practice. To achieve this, Kataoka and colleagues (2018)[35] recommend workplace assessment and workforce training and implementation tools that consistently incorporate trauma-informed principles. Trauma and resilience informed workforce development models should focus on reciprocal collaboration between academic centers, public service systems, and community partners (ie, community providers and residents), which is necessary to integrate culturally humble, evidence-based trauma and resilience strategies to promote mental health and reduce inequities in marginalized and underresourced communities.

THE DMH + UCLA PUBLIC PARTNERSHIP FOR WELLBEING: A FOUNDATION FOR IMPLEMENTING TRAUMA AND RESILIENCE INFORMED CARE

Similar to other large public mental health service systems, DMH faces many challenges to ensuring the mental health and well-being of diverse children, youth, and families disproportionately affected by adversity and trauma, including poverty and systemic racism. These services, from prevention through intensive treatment and recovery, are often undertaken in coordination with a complex array of child and family-serving systems (schools, child welfare, etc), community-based agencies, and larger community ecosystems (parks, libraries, etc).[36] Often marginalized and underresourced families experience structural barriers to mental health if there are not adequate employment protections, provision of housing, health care access, and strong safety nets, as well as the ongoing impact of exposure to trauma and adversity. Highly vulnerable youth are disproportionately served in mental health, child welfare, and juvenile justice settings and may face disruptions when moving between service systems. These adversities are often compounded when frontline providers in these often-stressed systems experience threats to their own personal and professional well-being due to burnout and moral distress. These challenges underscore the profound need for trauma-informed services for children, youth, and families in LA County, particularly for underresourced youth who face existing barriers to accessing mental health care.[37] Building a trauma and resilience informed community requires alignment of health, educational, and other service systems supporting youth and families.

In June 2018, DMH joined with UCLA to develop the DMH + UCLA PPFW, designed to leverage the strengths of these two public institutions to build a stronger and more resilient safety net in LA County. The PPFW includes the development of an internal DMH Strike Team (including individuals with lived and professional experiences with mental health implementation and system transformation) working alongside DMH leadership and UCLA faculty and staff to support collaborative communication and effective implementation. A core program of the PPFW, the DMH + UCLA Prevention Center of Excellence (Prevention COE) (wellbeing4la.org) was designed to specifically support the implementation of trauma and resilience informed practice across LA County departments and ecosystems. The Prevention COE was informed by the nationally recognized principles of trauma and resilience informed practice[27,38] as well as by extensive community, family, and other stakeholder engagement initiatives in LA County. In addition, the Prevention COE uses an ongoing community-partnered participatory approach to join with community partners, listen to community needs, and correspondingly codevelop and implement tailored training, coaching, and technical support to promote trauma and resilience informed services across DMH partnership agencies, including the LA County Office of Education, Department of Children and Family Services, Department of Human Resources, Department of Health Services, Probation Department, and Public Library, as well as community-based organizations, philanthropy, and other child well-being stakeholders. With a focus on building capacity, the Prevention COE provides a range of implementation and system transformation activities, including live training (in-person and virtual), asynchronous online learning, workforce well-being supports, population measurement and evaluation, policy and advocacy, cross-system communication, and program innovation.

To ensure that training topics relevant to providers and curricula are culturally humble, the Prevention COE begins each project with a community, family, and youth engagement process. Initial requests for support are drawn from a range of stakeholders, including professionals, county leadership, organizations, or community members. Potential topics are often discovered through engagement with stakeholders during activities and breakout groups at previous training. Listening sessions with community members help to better understand the need and possible strategies to leverage community strengths to meet that need. For example, while working with school-based mental health teams, it became clear that there was a need for educators to adapt strategies to engage students during the COVID-19 pandemic. A team of curriculum developers and trainers collaborated with school leaders, teachers, families, and mental health providers to coconstruct free and accessible virtual dialogue (online series "*Educators Overcoming Under Stress*"), virtual training, and other digital resources and toolkits (eg, increasing virtual student engagement, responding to systemic racism in the classroom, managing student, parent, and teacher anxiety). National experts joined to copresent with local professionals to address emerging science that could be contextualized to the specific experiences of residents in LA County.

The Prevention COE has anchored its training and professional development activities within a model of change that targets ecological outcomes (**Fig. 2**). This model

DMH + UCLA Prevention COE Model of Change

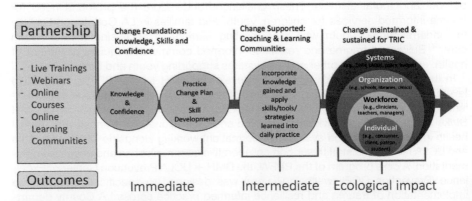

* TRIC: Trauma and Resilience Informed Care

Fig. 2. Prevention Center of Excellence model of change.

outlines the mechanisms through which positive foundations for change are established, supported, and maintained by service providers, community organizations, and ecosystems. Following a community-partnered participatory approach,[39] training curricula are developed in close partnership with community stakeholders, using a listening approach to use and customize evidence-based curricula as well as identify and share "practice-based evidence" to reflect a process of iterative learning through implementation.[40,41] All training and coaching curricula include attention to workforce well-being with skill-building and self-care to support individual and organizational resilience. Tailored assessment is conducted to better understand the unique stressors experienced by specific populations or workplaces, as well as the context for engagement of families, delivery of services, and opportunities for innovation.

Prevention COE trainings are designed to provide a foundation for supporting the longer-term goals of TRIC: improving outcomes for individuals (eg, improving client outcomes), workforce (eg, reducing burnout, turnover), naturally occurring community-based settings (eg, policy, procedure), and systems (eg, cost-effectiveness, funding). Consistent with the principles of trauma-informed care,[27] this partnership-driven approach leverages evidence-based educational tools to establish stigma-free learning environments, cultivate leadership and team skill sets, and support the overall well-being of peer and professional service providers.

The Prevention COE has been developed to align with and support sustainable implementation of prevention within LA County's ecosystems that is scientifically rigorous, innovative, as well as culturally humble. The Prevention COE uses a continuous quality improvement process in the development of training and implementation to provide consistent data monitoring and routine reporting to ensure that the Prevention COE can be responsive to emerging workforce development needs of LA County and remains harmonious with practices implemented by DMH. Educational tools and curricula help providers reduce re-traumatization, strengthen resilience, and improve the mental health and well-being of children, families, and adults within systems of care.

CORE PRINCIPLES AND ACTIVITIES FOR ESTABLISHING SIMILAR PARTNERSHIPS
Focus on Equity

One core principle of this partnership is to build equity for children, youth, and families using an ecological model, which outlines how the structural environment influences child development with individuals embedded in families, who are themselves embedded in schools and communities within larger policies driven by systemic racism and poverty.[42,43] This framework also recognizes that youth, families, and communities are critical collaborators in the identification, development, and implementation of programs and policies that can effectively support well-being.[27] Using a population health approach to the development of trauma-responsive systems, the PPFW has focused on building equity for children, youth, and families by highlighting areas of need, elevating youth and family voices, and leveraging community strengths. This partnership has also been developed to deepen an understanding of the ways that racial disparities and structural inequities have impacted community mental health and well-being as well as the services and resources available to children, youth, and families.[36]

Intentional and Ongoing Engagement

Increasingly, community-engaged and community-partnered approaches with diverse communities[44–46] have been recognized by the National Institutes of Health as effective in reducing health disparities.[44] By adopting a collaborative and community-partnered approach, the Prevention COE has been better positioned to promote mental health and well-being in the linguistically and culturally diverse communities in LA County. The inclusion of diverse perspectives from service providers, educators, administrators, families, researchers, and students strengthens the conceptual frameworks, implementation, and dissemination of preventive mental health strategies. This process is founded on valuing each stakeholder equally and honoring the diverse perspectives, skills, and strengths that each member brings to the collaboration. Using this community-partnered approach supports the adoption and integration of TRIC practices among community services and ecosystems because the strategies are authentically cocreated and informed by diverse stakeholders. Further, services become more responsive to the needs of diverse families and communities, and outreach efforts are better attuned to the ways that people prefer to engage mental health promotion and prevention.[27] Community champions and natural gatekeepers are engaged in the process as they are likely to be the most trusted source of information for many families. Authentic and sustained collaboration with key champions has been identified as an important strategy to increase trust in programs and implementation processes.[39]

Successful participatory-driven services depend upon active, intentional, and ongoing engagement with children, youth, and families. Community members are the best informants to help providers understand their challenges and strengths and the ways they prefer to receive services. Together, providers, researchers, and community members can best develop and deliver practices that focus on addressing needs in a manner that is culturally humble and responsive to diverse families.[47] Collaborating with children, youth, and families to describe variants of well-being across subgroups and contexts may be valuable to tailor services effectively. It is important, however, to realize that all communities have subgroups with a range of experience, backgrounds, and cultures, and thus programs must also realize and address multiple complexities.[39] Even well-developed services created from a participatory model must remain agile to adapt to emerging needs and styles in terms of what works, how it is best delivered, when is the optimal time, and for whom.

Continuous Mapping, Measurement, and Monitoring

In order to work effectively with the complex network of service systems that support community well-being, it is important to measure success and monitor quality. Service systems are dynamic and intricate in their structure and interconnected relationships, all with the goal of impacting communities beyond what any one system could do unilaterally.[48,49] As a result, methods of measurement and monitoring must be informed by and responsive to each component while it captures change across systems. A continuous quality improvement process is one in which outcomes are tracked with the goal of simultaneously measuring, informing, and adapting processes. For example, a training curriculum is never considered static or final in that it will always be customized for a new audience, adapted to accommodate emerging evidence and events, and modified to include strategies to better meet the needs of systems, agencies, and community members.

Consistent with the other core principles, measurement and monitoring strategies must be equitable, community-engaged, and sustainable. Investment in information infrastructures that support continuous quality improvement is needed to ensure the implementation of services that can adapt over time in response to emerging needs. Such an infrastructure provides a complex adaptive system with the flexibility to improve over time, providing decision-makers with useful information that allows them to make policies that are more equitable and driven by community needs and preferences and are simple and cost-effective enough to implement regularly consistent with a "learning community system."[50,51] Much of this work has been driven by the field of implementation science, which has a goal of closing the evidence-to-practice application gap.[52] Drawn from failures of successful evidence-based practice adoption, new processes have been developed to improve the translation from scientific study into practice and get scientifically sound strategies into the hands of the people who serve people directly.[53]

The adaptation, adoption, and implementation of evidence-informed strategies are done most successfully when it is done in partnership with delivery settings and practice organizations.[26] Thus, adherence to the core principle of mapping, measurement, and monitoring has both ensured that the Prevention COE is informed by emerging needs and monitored for accountability. This process has also assisted in effectively telling the story of the Prevention COE so that it is accountable to LA County stakeholders.

Sustainability

Sustainability reflects an organization's or system's capacity to deliver the benefits of empirically supported practices over time while both maintaining fidelity and being responsive to evolving needs.[40,41] In the Prevention COE, the foundations for sustainability have been developed in several ways that have been informed by implementation science. First, the academic community mental health partnership has developed foundational components of an implementation infrastructure that supports accessible interdisciplinary virtual training, coaching, and participatory learning communities. This infrastructure provides ongoing education and professional development for a diverse and geographically distributed workforce to engage in training and build community connections. As noted above, a culture and infrastructure to support sustainability are best achieved when service relevance and responsiveness are developed and maintained in partnership with communities. Making sure the organizational culture, policies, and procedures balance implementation fidelity with creative tailoring to cultural contexts supports the longevity of any new workplace practice. This also requires inclusiveness practices among leadership. As Nembhard and Edmonson (2006)[54] [(p961)] have described, models for inclusive leadership can apply to "organizations with cross-disciplinary teams, status diversity and a need for teams to continuously improve the services or products the organization produces." Given that the Prevention COE supports a network of complex and interlocking child and family serving service delivery systems, as well as community ecosystems, it has been important to focus on attention to leadership development in addition to staff learning in order to support sustainable change.

IMPLEMENTATION OF PRINCIPLES INTO PRACTICE: *DMH + UCLA WELLBEING FOR LA LEARNING CENTER*

A cornerstone of addressing the challenges of collaborative, evidence-based implementation support in a complex adaptive system such as LA County has been the development of a personalized learning management system that provides opportunities for interdisciplinary training, coaching, and learning communities. Diverse teams of learners can use the platform for synchronous and asynchronous education, professional development, and engagement to support implementation across county departments and ecosystems, from mental health, health care, schools, libraries, human resources, child welfare, juvenile justice, and other social service workforces, whether county service settings or community-based organizations.

Using the principles of human-centered design,[55] the learning management system has been developed and expanded in collaboration with community members. The learning platform personalizes content and engagement experiences for the user using machine learning and integrates qualitative and quantitative feedback using a continuous quality monitoring infrastructure to support the ongoing iteration of expanded content and platform configurations based on user experiences.

Launched just before the COVID-19 pandemic, the *DMH + UCLA Wellbeing Learning Center* (learn.wellbeing4LA.org) has demonstrated how a flexible, responsive learning platform can rapidly create a virtual learning environment that is responsive to emerging mental health needs and virtual relationships through teams of learners, which was particularly critical during the pandemic's remote work and educational environments. With more than 14,000 members of the county workforce enrolling in training in the first year of launch, the *Learning Center* provides personalized recommendations to bring more relevant and interesting content to each individual user, and specialized portals (such as for community peer workforce) create customized learning and certification pathways. Consistent with building an infrastructure to support engagement, equity, and sustainability, the *Learning Center* has created a range of virtual *Learning Communities* that bring together teams with the goals of fostering interaction, sharing knowledge, creative practice, providing engagement forums, developing resource libraries, sharing implementation support, and building relationships. The *Learning Center* also supports continuous monitoring and measurement that enable mapping of resources and activities based on population needs (for example, using public data metrics to monitor social vulnerability[56] as well as COVID-19 impact and providing dashboard-based decision-making insights to LA County decision-makers). This integrated dashboard provides detailed information about areas of highest needs, as well as real-time tracking deployment of training and implementation resources by zip code and supervisorial districts.

CONCLUSION

A public health response to build resilience and mitigate the impact of adversity and trauma in children and families requires a population-level approach across community ecosystems and service systems. Implementation science and participatory community approaches provide important insights to develop population-level trauma and resilience informed practices driven by a culture of continuous improvement. University-community partnerships that create a culture of reciprocal learning that honors lived experience and practice-based evidence can advance equity and well-being in marginalized and underresourced children, families, and communities.

For almost three years, the partnership of the LA County DMH and UCLA has led the creation of trauma and resilience informed community service services and ecosystems to support child, youth, and family well-being. Important lessons have been learned from this ongoing process. First, the partnership has had to be highly responsive to local contextual and cultural factors that affect mental health and well-being in families, including the disproportional impact of trauma, poverty, structural racism, health and educational inequities, food insecurity, inadequate housing and employment protections, and other adversities occurring without an adequate safety net. In addition, new and often unexpected factors will emerge. Most recently, our work has focused on supporting well-being during the time of the COVID-19 pandemic, national and local demonstrations in response to anti-Black racism, and political uncertainties. Organizational readiness, agility, and adaptability have been critical to providing continuity, responsivity, and sustainability during seemingly constant transitions.

Second, the partnership must bridge complex service systems and ecosystems. Leadership and providers from different child-serving systems (eg, education, health care, child welfare, and juvenile justice) have to be brought together to build shared knowledge across systems and to better understand the needs and experience of the youth and families with a focus on centering their experiences and trajectories, rather than a focus on the systems themselves. When organizations, leaders, and staff have worked together alongside families, the partnership has been able to advance trauma and resilience informed promotion and prevention services that reach children and families where they live.

Third, the partnership has leveraged both practice and academic expertise using an equitable approach that aims to reduce silos and develop shared language and collaborative practices. When strong academic and public partnerships are valued, it creates a culture of reciprocal learning that honors lived experience and practice-based evidence. Further, approaches such as the *Wellbeing for LA Learning Center Learning Communities* can initiate, grow, and sustain these partnerships while supporting the practical application of knowledge, skills, and collaborative care.

Building successful partnerships is not without its challenges. Collaboration requires patience, strategic thinking, deliberate coconstruction of resources, innovative engagement strategies, and continuous adaptation. Nevertheless, long-term benefits are conferred through creating community services, and ecosystems that support the well being of children, youth, and families throughout their lifespans to improve public health are monumental.

DISCLOSURE

We acknowledge this article reflects activities of the public partnership between Los Angeles County Department of Mental Health and UCLA which is supported by LAC DMH Contract MH270001 to UCLA.

REFERENCES

1. Evans GW, Li D, Whipple SS. Cumulative risk and child development. Psychol Bull 2013;139(6):1342–96.
2. Felitti VJ, Anda RF, Nordenberg D, et al. Relationship of childhood abuse and household dysfunction to many of the leading causes of death in adults. The Adverse Childhood Experiences (ACE) Study. Am J Prev Med 1998;14(4): 245–58.
3. CDC. About the CDC-kaiser ACE study 2019. Available at: https://www.cdc.gov/violenceprevention/aces/about.html. Accessed May 13, 2021.
4. Dube SR, Felitti VJ, Dong M, et al. The impact of adverse childhood experiences on health problems: evidence from four birth cohorts dating back to 1900. Prev Med 2003;37(3):268–77.
5. Merrick MT, Ford DC, Ports KA, et al. Prevalence of adverse childhood experiences from the 2011-2014 behavioral risk factor surveillance system in 23 states. JAMA Pediatr 2018;172(11):1038.
6. Anda RF, Felitti VJ, Bremner JD, et al. The enduring effects of abuse and related adverse experiences in childhood. Eur Arch Psychiatry Clin Neurosci 2006; 256(3):174–86.

7. Juster R-P, McEwen BS, Lupien SJ. Allostatic load biomarkers of chronic stress and impact on health and cognition. Neurosci Biobehav Rev 2010;35(1):2–16.

8. Elias A, Paradies Y. Estimating the mental health costs of racial discrimination. BMC Public Health 2016;16(1):1205.

9. Heard-Garris NJ, Cale M, Camaj L, et al. Transmitting Trauma: a systematic review of vicarious racism and child health. Soc Sci Med 2018;199:230–40.

10. Kumar M, Fonagy P. Differential effects of exposure to social violence and natural disaster on children's mental health. J Trauma Stress 2013;26(6):695–702.

11. Dubé C, Gagné M-H, Clément M-È, et al. Community violence and associated psychological problems among adolescents in the General population. J Child Adolesc Trauma 2018;11(4):411–20.

12. Centers for Disease Control and Prevention. Adverse childhood experiences (ACEs). 2021. Available at: https://www.cdc.gov/violenceprevention/aces/index.html. Accessed May 14, 2021.

13. Berkes F, Ross H. Community resilience: toward an integrated approach. Soc Nat Resour 2013;26(1):5–20.

14. Menschner C, Maul. Key ingredients for trauma-informed care implementation. Center for Health Care Strategies; 2016. Available at: https://www.chcs.org/resource/key-ingredients-for-successful-trauma-informed-care-implementation/. Accessed May 14, 2021.

15. The National Child Traumatic Stress Network. What is a trauma-informed child and family service system? 2016. Available at: https://www.nctsn.org/resources/what-trauma-informed-child-and-family-service-system. Accessed May 13, 2021.

16. Hoge MA, Morris JA, Stuart GW, et al. A national action plan for workforce development in behavioral health. Psychiatr Serv 2009;60(7):883–7.

17. Masten AS. Resilience theory and research on children and families: past, present, and promise. J Fam Theor Rev 2018;10(1):12–31.

18. Sroufe LA. Psychopathology as an outcome of development. Dev Psychopathol 1997;9(2):251–68.

19. National Research Council (US) and Institute of Medicine (US) Committee on the prevention of mental disorders and substance abuse among children, youth, and young adults: research advances and promising interventions. In: O'Connell ME, Boat T, Warner KE, editors. Preventing mental, emotional, and behavioral disorders among young people: progress and possibilities. National Academies Press (US); 2009. Available at: http://www.ncbi.nlm.nih.gov/books/NBK32775/. Accessed May 13, 2021.

20. Spoth R. Translating family-focused prevention science into effective practice: toward a translational impact paradigm. Curr Dir Psychol Sci 2008;17(6):415–21.

21. Lester P. The time has come: integrating trauma-informed prevention within systems of care. In: Research presentation at the 65th annual American academy of child and adolescent psychiatry, Seattle, Washington. 2018. Available at: https://www.jaacap.org/article/S0890-8567(18)31363-7/fulltext. Accessed May 13, 2021.

22. National Research Council (US) and Institute of Medicine (US). Committee on depression, parenting practices, and the healthy development of children. In: England MJ, Sim LJ, editors. Depression in parents, parenting, and children: opportunities to improve identification, treatment, and prevention. National Academies Press (US); 2009. http://www.ncbi.nlm.nih.gov/books/NBK215117/. Accessed May 14, 2021.

23. Narayan AJ, Lieberman AF, Masten AS. Intergenerational transmission and prevention of adverse childhood experiences (ACEs). Clin Psychol Rev 2021;85: 101997.
24. Institute of Medicine (US) Committee on prevention of mental disorders. In: Mrazek PJ, Haggerty RJ, editors. Reducing risks for mental disorders: frontiers for preventive intervention research. National Academies Press (US); 1994. Available at: http://www.ncbi.nlm.nih.gov/books/NBK236319/. Accessed May 13, 2021.
25. National Academies of Sciences E. Preventing bullying through science, policy, and practice 2016. https://doi.org/10.17226/23482.
26. National Academies of Sciences E. Strengthening the military family readiness system for a changing American society 2019. https://doi.org/10.17226/25380.
27. Substance Abuse and Mental Health Services Administration. SAMHSA's concept of trauma and guidance for a trauma-informed approach. National Institute of Corrections; 2014. Available at: https://nicic.gov/samhsas-concept-trauma-and-guidance-trauma-informed-approach. Accessed May 13, 2021.
28. Elliott DE, Bjelajac P, Fallot RD, et al. Trauma-informed or trauma-denied: principles and implementation of trauma-informed services for women. J Community Psychol 2005;33(4):461–77.
29. Masten AS. Global perspectives on resilience in children and youth. Child Dev 2014;85(1):6–20.
30. Luthar SS, Cicchetti D. The construct of resilience: implications for interventions and social policies. Dev Psychopathol 2000;12(4):857–85.
31. Masten AS, Hubbard JJ, Gest SD, et al. Competence in the context of adversity: pathways to resilience and maladaptation from childhood to late adolescence. Dev Psychopathol 1999;11(1):143–69.
32. Wyman PA, Cowen EL, Work WC, et al. Caregiving and developmental factors Differentiating young at-risk urban children showing resilient versus stress-affected outcomes: a replication and extension. Child Dev 1999;70(3):645–59.
33. Masten AS. Resilience from a developmental systems perspective. World Psychiatry 2019;18(1):101–2.
34. Magis K. Community resilience: an indicator of social sustainability. Soc Nat Resour 2010;23(5):401–16.
35. Kataoka SH, Vona P, Acuna A, et al. Applying a trauma informed school systems approach: examples from school community-academic partnerships. Ethn Dis 2018;28(Suppl 2):417–26.
36. Ijadi-Maghsoodi R, Harrison D, Kelman A, et al. Leveraging a public-public partnership in Los Angeles County to address COVID-19 for children, youth, and families in underresourced communities. Psychol Trauma Theor Res Pract Policy 2020;12(5):457–60.
37. Kataoka SH, Zhang L, Wells KB. Unmet need for mental health care among U.S. Children: variation by ethnicity and insurance status. Am J Psychiatry 2002; 159(9):1548–55.
38. Centers for Disease Control and Prevention. Infographic: 6 guiding principles to a trauma-informed approach. 2020. Available at: https://www.cdc.gov/cpr/infographics/6_principles_trauma_info.htm. Accessed May 13, 2021.
39. Wallerstein N, Duran B. Community-based participatory research contributions to intervention research: the intersection of science and practice to improve health equity. Am J Public Health 2010;100(Suppl 1):S40–6.
40. Chambers DA, Norton WE. The adaptome: advancing the science of intervention adaptation. Am J Prev Med 2016;51(4 Suppl 2):S124–31.

41. Brownson RC, Fielding JE, Green LW. Building capacity for evidence-based public health: reconciling the pulls of practice and the push of research. Annu Rev Public Health 2018;39:27–53.
42. Bronfenbrenner U. The ecology of human development: experiments by nature and design. Cambridge (MA): Harvard University Press; 1979.
43. Bronfenbrenner U, Ceci SJ. Nature-nurture reconceptualized in developmental perspective: a bioecological model. Psychol Rev 1994;101(4):568–86.
44. Wallerstein NB, Duran B. Using community-based participatory research to address health disparities. Health Promot Pract 2006;7(3):312–23.
45. Blumenthal DS. Is community-based participatory research possible? Am J Prev Med 2011;40(3):386–9.
46. Trickett EJ, Beehler S, Deutsch C, et al. Advancing the science of community-level interventions. Am J Public Health 2011;101(8):1410–9.
47. Lekas H-M, Pahl K, Fuller Lewis C. Rethinking cultural competence: shifting to cultural humility. Health Serv Insights 2020;13:1–4.
48. Ellis B, Herbert S. Complex adaptive systems (CAS): an overview of key elements, characteristics and application to management theory. J Innov Health Inform 2011;19(1):33–7.
49. Spivey MJ. Discovery in complex adaptive systems. Cogn Syst Res 2018;51: 40–55.
50. Institute of Medicine (US). In: Grossmann C, Powers B, McGinnis JM, editors. Digital infrastructure for the learning health system: the foundation for continuous improvement in health and health care: workshop series summary. National Academies Press (US); 2011. Available at: http://www.ncbi.nlm.nih.gov/books/NBK83569/. Accessed May 13, 2021.
51. Medicine I of. Best care at lower cost: the path to continuously learning health care in America 2012. https://doi.org/10.17226/13444.
52. Proctor EK, Landsverk J, Aarons G, et al. Implementation research in mental health services: an emerging science with conceptual, methodological, and training challenges. Adm Policy Ment Health 2009;36(1):24–34.
53. Kelly B. Implementing implementation science: reviewing the quest to develop methods and frameworks for effective implementation. J Neurol Psychol 2013; 1(1):5.
54. Nembhard IM, Edmondson AC. Making it safe: the effects of leader inclusiveness and professional status on psychological safety and improvement efforts in health care teams. J Organ Behav 2006;27(7):941–66.
55. Cooley M. Human-centred systems. In: Rosenbrock H, editor. *Designing human-centred technology: a cross-disciplinary project in computer-aided manufacturing.* The springer series on artificial intelligence and society. Springer; 1989. p. 133–43.
56. CDC/ATSDR's social vulnerability index (SVI). 2021. Available at: https://www.atsdr.cdc.gov/placeandhealth/svi/index.html. Accessed May 13, 2021.

Collaboration with Schools and School-Based Health Centers

Erika Ryst, MD[a],*, Shashank V. Joshi, MD[b,c]

KEYWORDS

- School-based mental health • Delivery of health care • Integrated care models
- Consultation liaison • Collaborative • Well-being in youth • Health promotion

KEY POINTS

- As models of school-based health care have evolved, increasing attention has been paid to the important role of mental health delivered in school settings.
- School-based mental health offers increased access to care, increased acceptability, decreased stigma, removal of transportation barriers, affordability, and direct observation in the school setting.
- Studies of school-based health services demonstrate positive outcomes in physical health, mental health and educational achievement.
- Newer models of school-based mental health provide prevention and a continuum of services across collaborative systems of community and school-based health.
- The field of school-based mental health offers opportunities for systems change, mental health promotion, suicide prevention, population health, health care equity and integrated service delivery.

INTRODUCTION

Rates of youth mental health problems approach 20%,[1] yet most children and teens with these problems do not access help.[2] The current system of care for youth mental health is fragmented, inaccessible to many (including the most vulnerable youth), and inefficient. Furthermore, the ongoing stigma regarding mental health disorders prevents many youth from seeking help.[3]

Schools represent a major access point for mental health services. As the saying goes, "school is where the children are", and school personnel have a unique

[a] Nevada Center for Excellence in Disabilities, College of Education and Human Development, University of Nevada, Reno, 4090 William J. Raggio Building, 1664 N. Virginia Street, Suite 4090, Mail Stop: 285, Reno, NV 89557, USA; [b] Stanford University, Stanford, CA, USA; [c] Lucile Packard Children's Hospital @ Stanford, 401 Quarry Road, Stanford, CA 94305-5719, USA
* Corresponding author.
E-mail address: eryst@med.unr.edu

Child Adolesc Psychiatric Clin N Am 30 (2021) 751–765
https://doi.org/10.1016/j.chc.2021.07.004
1056-4993/21/© 2021 Elsevier Inc. All rights reserved.

childpsych.theclinics.com

opportunity to identify and help children suffering from problems with mental health. By locating mental health services within schools, many more children can access needed services in the familiar and comfortable environment of school. In fact, families perceive school-based mental health care services as a needed support that can overcome barriers to service access.[4] Additional benefits for locating mental health care services within schools include the ability for direct observation of challenging behaviors and the possibility of integrating mental health care interventions within a comprehensive, public health framework.[5]

The exciting expansion of child mental health services within schools offer new and innovative practice opportunities for child and adolescent psychiatrists. Working within and together with school communities, child and adolescent psychiatrists can influence new mental health service delivery models that have the potential to reach greater numbers of youth, to provide earlier intervention, and to reduce health care disparities. This article will introduce the historical context, delivery models, key terminology, and current evidence base supporting school-based mental health. Finally, by presenting specific examples of how child and adolescent psychiatrists can provide direct service, consultation, or technical assistance to schools, the authors hope to inspire child and adolescent psychiatrists to join the growing field of school-based mental health.

HISTORY

The history of school-based health and mental health services dates back to the early 1900s, when school-based nurses were first introduced. However, it was not until the late 1960s that efforts to link health care and education resulted in the first school-based health centers (SBHCs). The first SBHCs were originally funded by the American Academy of Pediatrics Community Access to Child Health Grants and federal Title X Family Planning Program funds and were primarily aimed toward contraception and preventing teenage pregnancy. By 1985, there were 31 SBHCs across 18 urban areas in the United States, and by 1998 to 1999, there were 1135 SBHCs located in 45 states. This rapid expansion of SBHCs was fueled by a growing recognition that access to care could be improved by locating services in school, as well as a growing national interest in integrating services.[5–9] While initial SBHC efforts largely focused on primary care rather than mental health, by the 1990s, interest in school mental health resulted in federal funding of two national school mental health centers (the National Center for School Mental Health [NCSMH] based at the University of Maryland and the Center for School Mental Health at the University of California, Los Angeles). These two centers have been instrumental in promoting, researching, and providing technical assistance on school mental health and remain pivotal to the field of school mental health today. Increasing emphasis on the importance of mental health has also led most SBHCs (65%) to include mental health services within their delivery model.[10]

Heightened interest and awareness about the need for school-based mental health services continued through the 2000s, galvanized unfortunately by school shootings such as the 2012 Newtown, Connecticut, school shooting. In response to these school shootings, President Obama released his "Now is the Time" presidential plan to protect children and communities by reducing gun violence. Through this initiative, $40 million dollars was allocated to SAMHSA to fund pilot demonstration school-based mental health programs in 20 states ("Project AWARE—Advancing Wellness and Resilience in Education"). The Project AWARE program is one of several recent federal funding projects that have worked to advance school-based mental health.[11] Other recent federally funded projects of note include supplemental funding to address the need for increased school-based mental health services that were awarded to the Mental Health Technology Transfer Center Network in August of 2018 and establishment of the National Center on Safe Supportive Learning Environments starting in 2012. As school mental health becomes an even more salient issue as a result of widespread school closures necessitated by the COVID-19 pandemic, it is likely that even more attention and funding opportunities will arise in the field of school-based mental health. Please see **Table 1** for a timeline of dates associated with important events in the evolution of school-based health and mental health care.

DEFINITIONS AND MODELS OF SCHOOL-BASED HEALTH AND MENTAL HEALTH

Several different terms have been used to describe models of school-based health and mental health. These differences in terminology reflect the variability of school-based service delivery models, as well as a gradual evolution toward more comprehensive and public health–based models. Please see **Table 2** for a listing of the more common terms used to describe the various models.

As described in the History section, the original delivery of school-based health services has evolved over time into increasingly more integrated and comprehensive systems of service. While SBHCs do not have to include a mental health component, as of the most recent national school-based health care census, most SBHCs (65%) now include behavioral health.[10] The growing recognition of the importance of mental health for youth, as well as the fact that most SBHC adolescent visits are for substance abuse or mental health reasons, likely has contributed to this change.[22] However, as pointed out by Larson and colleagues, the mental health care delivered within SBHCs does not necessarily equate to comprehensive mental health care.[23] Similarly, while most schools across the country provide some form of school-based mental health services, many of these programs exist in silos and lack integration with other systems.[17]

To improve the overall system of mental health care within schools, recent national efforts have encouraged the development of Comprehensive School Mental Health Systems (CSMHS). The NCSMH at the University of Maryland School of Medicine is one of the organizations at the forefront of these efforts (http://www.schoolmentalhealth.org). Originally founded in 1995, the NCSMH receives core funding from the Health Resources and Services Administration, Maternal and Child Health Bureau, to provide technical assistance and training for the advancement of research, training, policy, and practice in school mental health. As part of its core mission, the NCSMH promotes CSMHS through a variety of trainings, technical assistance, and strategic initiatives. The CSMHS approach eclipses more traditional approaches to school-based mental health care by including prevention, positive school climate, collaboration (between all stakeholders—school, community providers, parents, students, and families), social determinants of health, and public policy within an integrated and comprehensive framework and therefore represents greater potential for innovative system change. The new "School Wellness Center" moniker for SBHCs reflects this evolutionary movement toward more integrated, comprehensive, and preventative approaches. **Fig. 1** visually represents the interconnected subsystems involved in CSMHS.

CURRENT EVIDENCE

A body of evidence currently exists that supports the delivery of school-based health and mental health care services. First, several studies indicate positive outcomes in

Table 1
Timeline of important events in the evolution of school-based health and mental health care

Time Period	Events
Early 1900s	Start of the school nurse model
Late 1960s	First school-based health centers (SBHCs) in urban areas
1985	First National School-Based Health Care Census identifies 31 SBHCs in 18 urban sites.
1990	Medicaid expansion helps to increase SBHC sustainability; increased federal interest in integrated services
1995	Congress earmarks community health center funds for SBHCs; HRSA-MCHB funds two national centers on school mental health, one based at the University of Maryland and the other at the University of California, Los Angeles.
1998–99	National School-Based Health Care Census identifies 1135 SBHCs (10-fold increase over a decade).
2000	SBHCs are identified as eligible to receive new federal funding for community health centers.
2003	The President's New Freedom Commission on Mental Health explicitly recommends to improve and expand school mental health programs.
2004	The American Academy of Pediatrics publishes a policy statement on School-Based Mental Health Services; the National Research Council and Institute of Medicine identifies children's education as a health outcome.
2010	The Patient Protection and Affordable Care Act authorizes $200 million to increase the capacity of SBHCs
2013	President Obama releases his "Now is the Time" presidential plan to protect our children and communities by reducing gun violence. Through this initiative, $15 million was allocated for Youth Mental Health First Aid training, and $40 million was awarded by SAMHSA to 20 states to develop school-based mental health demonstration pilot projects
2014	The CDC launches the "Whole School, Whole Community, Whole Child Model" that builds on the earlier "Coordinated School Health" approach by expanding components that include mental health and community engagement.
2019	The National Center for School Mental Health publishes: "Advancing Comprehensive School Mental Health Together: Guidance for the Field"
2020–2021	National school closures due to the COVID-19 pandemic; increasing awareness and concern regarding youth mental health and impact on schools.

both health and education as a result of SBHCs. From a health perspective, SBHCs have been shown to increase immunization rates, decrease hospitalizations and emergency room visits for chronic medical conditions, reduce rates of teenage pregnancy, and increase adolescent contraceptive use.[8,9,24,25] SBHCs also significantly impact mental health outcomes. For example, in one study, students receiving SBHC mental health services showed a significant decline in depression and reduced suicidal ideation.[26] Studies have also shown reduced rates of cigarette and marijuana use in students at schools with SBHCs compared with students at schools without SBHCs.[27] Mental health visits at SBHCs are most often related to pregnancy, sexuality, depression, suicidal ideation, conflict, and violence. Importantly, mental health services in SBHCs increase access to mental health care that adolescents are unlikely to receive

Table 2 Key terms related to school-based health and mental health	
School-based health services	This is a very broad term that covers preventative, acute, and emergency health services, care coordination, and chronic disease management provided by the school and delivered by qualified professionals such as school nurses, nurse practitioners, dentists, health educators, physicians, physician assistant, and allied health personnel.[12]
School-based health center (SBHC)	A specific type of school-based health service that brings together the health and education sectors to provide comprehensive medical care and referrals and serve as a medical home. There are four types of SBHC delivery models: traditional (located on school sites), school-linked (located near to and linked to a school site), mobile (services provided in a mobile vehicle such as a van), and telehealth exclusive (services only provided to school via telehealth). Mental health may or may not be included in this service delivery model.[13–15]
School-based mental health (SBMH)	Defined by Kones and Hoagwood as "any program, intervention, or strategy applied in a school setting that was specifically designed to influence students' emotional, behavioral, and/or social functioning.[16]" Core principles include services occurring in a school building, incorporating an array of services, and requiring school and community partnerships.[5] Generally delivery models either use school district personnel only to deliver the services, combine school personnel with community providers for service delivery, or coordinate referrals to outside community providers to deliver specific mental health services.[17]
Comprehensive School Mental Health Systems (CSMHS)	According to the National Center for School Mental Health, CSMHS "provide a full array of tiered supports and services that promote positive school climate, social and emotional learning, and mental health and well-being, while reducing the prevalence and severity of mental illness and substance use. CSMHS are built on a strong foundation of district and school professionals... in strategic collaboration with students, families,

(continued on next page)

Table 2 (continued)	
	and community health and mental health partners. These systems also assess and address the social, political, and environmental structures, including public policies and social norms, that influence mental health outcomes."[18]
Multi-Tiered Systems of Support (MTSS)	MTSS is a framework designed to improve outcomes for all students by using data-based decision-making to match students with evidence-based practices. Services are provided along a continuum ranging from Tier 1 (universal prevention for all) to Tier 2 (targeted intervention for some) to Tier 3 (intensive, individualized intervention for few).[19]
Positive Behavioral Interventions and Supports (PBIS)	PBIS is an evidence-based, three-tiered framework that uses the MTSS model to support positive behaviors in schools.
Interconnected Systems Framework (ISF)	ISF is a framework developed by leaders in the PBIS and mental health field to provide guidance on the integration of mental health and PBIS in schools[20]
School Wellness Centers	A new name for SBHCs that aim to expand the traditional mission of SBHCs to include population health, preventative services, health promotion, education, and health care for students, families, and the community.[21]

outside of school. One study found that adolescents were 21 times more likely to use mental health services in SBHCs than to use community-based clinics.[28]

While educational outcomes related to the delivery of school-based health and mental health care services are harder to study, there is also evidence of favorable outcomes in this domain. SBHCs have been found to be associated with increases in both school attendance, grade point average, and school connectedness.[8,9,29] Interestingly, one such study found that increases in attendance and grade point average were more strongly associated with mental health care service use.[25,29] SBHC use may also reduce high school dropout rates.[25]

A secondary analysis of the cross-sectional School-Based Health Alliance Census School Year 2010 to 2011 Report examined characteristic differences between SBHCs with and without mental health care providers.[23] This study found that 70% of SBHCs offered mental health care services. SBHCs with more resources, more students, a longer history, and state funding were more likely to offer mental health services. Furthermore, compared with SBHCs without a mental health care provider, SBHCs with a mental health care provider offered a broader range of services such as crisis intervention, case management, classroom behavior and

Exhibit 31

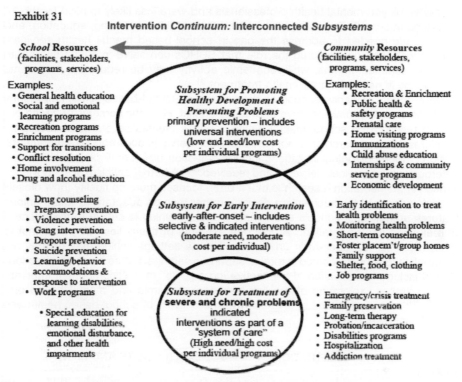

Intervention *Continuum:* Interconnected *Subsystems*

School **Resources**
(facilities, stakeholders,
programs, services)

Examples:
• General health education
• Social and emotional
learning programs
• Recreation programs
• Enrichment programs
• Support for transitions
• Conflict resolution
• Home involvement
• Drug and alcohol education

• Drug counseling
• Pregnancy prevention
• Violence prevention
• Gang intervention
• Dropout prevention
• Suicide prevention
• Learning/behavior
accommodations &
response to intervention
• Work programs

• Special education for
learning disabilities,
emotional disturbance,
and other health
impairments

*Subsystem for Promoting
Healthy Development &
Preventing Problems*
primary prevention – includes
universal interventions
(low end need/low cost
per individual programs)

Subsystem for Early Intervention
early-after-onset – includes
selective & indicated interventions
(moderate need, moderate
cost per individual)

Subsystem for Treatment of
severe and chronic problems
indicated
interventions as part of a
"system of care"
(High need/high cost
per individual programs)

Community **Resources**
(facilities, stakeholders,
programs, services)

Examples:
• Recreation & Enrichment
• Public health &
safety programs
• Prenatal care
• Home visiting programs
• Immunizations
• Child abuse education
• Internships & community
service programs
• Economic development

• Early identification to treat
health problems
• Monitoring health problems
• Short-term counseling
• Foster placem't/group homes
• Family support
• Shelter, food, clothing
• Job programs

• Emergency/crisis treatment
• Family preservation
• Long-term therapy
• Probation/incarceration
• Disabilities programs
• Hospitalization
• Addiction treatment

Fig. 1. Interconnected Subsystems in Comprehensive School Mental Health Systems (CSMHS). (Howard Adelman & Linda Taylor (2021). Embedding Mental Health as Schools Change. Available at http://smhp.psych.ucla.edu/barriersbook.pdf.)

learning support, peer mediation, health promotion, and prescription of mental health medications.

While SBHCs represent one possible integrated service delivery model for mental health, the reality is that less than 10% of schools across the country have access to SBHCs; at the same time, child mental health needs are great, access to community mental health resources is limited, and most children with mental health problems do not get treatment. While schools provide a variety of child mental health services, there is growing recognition that the current school-based mental health services are not enough, and educators are increasingly seeking to expand school-based mental health services.[30]

To map the landscape of school-based mental health service delivery, a recent study analyzed school mental health services data from the US Department of Education, National Center for Education Statistics, 2015 to 2016 School Survey on Crime and Safety.[17] On this survey, nearly 50% of schools reported providing treatment for mental health disorders outside of school by a school-funded professional. In contrast, less than 40% of schools provided treatment at school by either a school-employed or school-funded mental health professional. The major limitation reported by schools in providing mental health services was inadequate funding (41.6%); the second greatest limitation was inadequate access to mental health professionals (23.3%). Rural schools were statistically significantly less likely to have access to in-school employed mental health professionals and were less likely to have treatment programs at school. The authors concluded that additional funding, education, and services are needed to address the gap in school-based mental health services. Recent work has underscored the role that SBHCs can serve in supporting youth over the summer months, while academic activity may be reduced but students may still be in need of mental health treatment.[31]

While current evidence supporting the delivery of school-based health and mental health services is promising, several limitations exist. First, the community-based nature of research on school mental health services creates several methodological problems. Most research on school mental health services does not use experimental design.[32] Methodological limitations include selection bias, small sample sizes, and heterogeneity of services delivered and received.[8,24] A further criticism of school intervention implementation research is that it often focuses more on fidelity (how closely schools adhere to the intervention design), rather than on adaptations to the unique features of individual schools and school systems, which is critical to the success of real-world implementation.[8] A concrete example of this is lies in the fact that to date, most SBHCs operate in urban, low-income settings, which may or may not extrapolate to schools located in rural or suburban settings. Future research directions should include identification of the "active ingredients" of multicomponent interventions,[32] further exploration of the link between academic and mental health outcomes,[6,8] and applications of telehealth to the delivery of school-based health and mental health services.[6,33]

CHALLENGES IN IMPLEMENTATION OF SCHOOL-BASED HEALTH AND MENTAL HEALTH

In order to achieve the vision of fully integrated and CSMHS, several barriers and challenges must be overcome. One of the greatest challenges to date has been scarcity of funding for school-based mental health services. While schools and SBHCs are able to bill insurance for some services, other critical aspects of CSMHS such as interdisciplinary team meetings are not eligible for reimbursement.[9,34] The current COVID-19 pandemic and its consequences may actually help in this regard, as the U.S. federal government has specified school mental health as a target for the use of COVID relief funds.

A second challenge relates to mental health workforce demands. School-based mental health providers such as school counselors, school psychologists, and school social workers are often already overwhelmed with unmanageably large caseloads. "Opening the floodgates" by increasing mental health access through SBHCs and CSMHS will put increased workforce demand on a system that is already stressed. This problem surfaces in research findings such as that of Walter and colleagues, who found that despite the provision of multitiered mental health services through a hospital-school partnership, there was limited program reach.[32] Specifically, only 21% of the student population received preventative services (while ideally 100% of students would receive prevention), and only 2% of the student population received clinical services (while estimates indicate that at least 10% of students have mental health needs). The evaluators of this program also found that only one-tenth of the school staff believed that the schools had sufficient mental health resources.[32]

Finally, and perhaps most importantly, embedding mental health services in schools requires substantial system change, which is always fraught with challenge and resistance. Advocates for school mental health need to invest significant time in achieving school staff buy-in. Traditionally the mission of schools has been to promote academic achievement, and many educators still see student mental health as an un-related or secondary priority. Existing school mental health systems are often "ad-hoc" siloed and seen as a "support" rather than a primary service.[34] More research on the linkage between mental health and academic outcomes will be critical to convince educators of how CSMHS can benefit their core academic mission.

Even with school system buy-in, much work still needs to happen to integrate educational and medical systems. The educational and medical systems each have their own structures, vocabulary, regulations, and priorities which do not always align. A simple example of this is the problem of how to reconcile differences in legislation related to patient or student confidentiality (called "HIPPA" (the Health Insurance Portability and Accountability Act) on the medical side, and "FERPA" (the Family Educational Rights and Privacy Act) on the educational side). While the aims of legis-lation governing HIPPA and FERPA are similar, differences in regulation and imple-mentation can create barriers to the sharing of student information across the medical and educational systems. Overcoming these types of silos and barriers will be critical to the successful integration of the two systems.

ROLE OF THE CHILD AND ADOLESCENT PSYCHIATRIST IN SCHOOL COLLABORATION

Increasing awareness of the importance of youth mental health, the impact of youth mental health on school outcomes such as absenteeism and graduation rates, and newer models of CSMHS provides a unique opportunity for child and adolescent psy-chiatrists to become involved in school consultation. **Table 3** lists a variety of ways in which child and adolescent psychiatrists can provide such consultation.

Recent reviews have highlighted the role that psychiatrists can play in implementing programs that can promote literacy about mental health, reduce mental health stigma, and prevent suicide. Additionally, child and adolescent psychiatrists are well-positioned to collaborate with teachers to be "experts" for one another regarding the mental health of specific students.[35,36]

Successful child psychiatrist school consultation requires additional compe-tencies and skills beyond those necessary for standard office-based clinical care. At a minimum, the child psychiatrist school consultant will need to use knowledge and skills in each of the following domains: (1) consultation strategies (such as how to identify the consultation question, clarifying boundaries of the consultation role, and empowering the consultee); (2) special education law and the structure of schools; (3) specific school-based interventions and accommodations for com-mon mental disorders such as Attention-deficit/hyperactivity disorder (ADHD), pedi-atric anxiety, and depression; (4) evidence-based mental health interventions in schools such as Cognitive Behavioral Intervention for Trauma in Schools; (5) school threat assessment and crisis response (for example, when a student dies by suicide); and (6) systems thinking, such as appreciating the role of resistance to change when new interventions are introduced.[37,38] While training on most of these competencies is provided during child and adolescent psychiatry fellowship, for those who desire a refresher or more in-depth knowledge, multiple resources are available. Three web-sites in particular that provide a wealth of knowledge include the school mental health resource page of the Mental Health Transfer Technology website (https://mhttcnetwork.org/centers/global-mhttc/school-mental-health-resources), the Na-tional Center for School Mental Health website (http://www.schoolmentalhealth.org), and the Center for Mental Health in Schools at UCLA website (http://www.smhp.psych.ucla.edu).

Table 3
Ways in which child and adolescent psychiatrists (CAPs) may support school-based mental health

Type	Description	Examples
Direct service	The CAP provides a direct clinical service to either students or school staff. Services may be delivered at the school site, via telehealth, or at the CAP's office. The school may pay the CAP directly for the service, or the CAP or school may bill insurance. Alternatively, the CAP may be employed by an SBHC, children's hospital, or university.	• The CAP contracts with the school to provide child psychiatry evaluation and management of students referred to the CAP by the school. Releases of information are in place to allow for bidirectional communication between the CAP and the school. Telehealth can be a convenient way to deliver service, but the telehealth visit must be facilitated at the school site by school staff. • The CAP contracts with the school district to provide one-time, comprehensive school-based child psychiatry evaluations to provide both school-based and community-based recommendations. Typically such an evaluation includes review of school records, meeting with the school team, parent interview, school observation of the child, and child interview. The school team may then incorporate recommendations into the child's Individualized Education Plan (IEP). If needed, the CAP can facilitate community-based referrals. • The CAP contracts with the school to provide group psychotherapy interventions at the school, or to provide supervision of school-based mental health professionals in the delivery of school-based mental health interventions (such as Cognitive Behavioral Intervention for Trauma in Schools, CBITS).
Consultation	The CAP provides indirect support of school professionals to promote school-based mental health. Payment is usually in the form of compensation by the school as an hourly rate or portion of the CAP's full-time equivalent (FTE).	• The CAP participates in multidisciplinary school team meetings (such as ISF teams) to review school-wide academic and behavior data, community data, and universal mental health screening assessment

(continued on next page)

Table 3 (continued)		
Type	**Description**	**Examples**
		data to inform school mental health service delivery planning.
		• The CAP, together with school-based mental health professionals such as school psychologists and school counselors, works to promote mental health awareness among students, school staff, and parents. Resources to help the CAP and schools with this task include the National School Mental Health Curriculum (https://mhttcnetwork.org/centers/global-mhttc/national-smh-curriculum) and the evidence-based program Youth Mental Health First Aid (https://www.mentalhealthfirstaid.org/population-focused-modules/youth/).
		• The CAP provides education (such as virtual Zoom training sessions) on desired mental health topics for school staff or parent groups
		• The CAP provides training to school staff on evidence-based practices (such as Trauma-Informed Care) to expand the school staff capacity to deliver such practices.
		• The CAP provides informal case consultation to school teams on challenging cases—either independently, or together with an interdisciplinary team. The ECHO (Extending Community Healthcare Outcomes) format lends itself well to this type of interdisciplinary case consultation and provision of case-based recommendations within a professional learning community (https://hsc.unm.edu/echo/)
		• The CAP supports well-being of school personnel by either providing informal support, for example, by leading a peer supervision group of school-based mental health professionals, or by providing

(continued on next page)

Table 3 *(continued)*		
Type	Description	Examples
		formal classes on teacher wellbeing (such as the WISE Teacher Well-being Workbook by Jeff Bostic, M.D., Ed.D).
Technical assistance	The CAP provides expertise on solving school problems at a systems level by addressing school or district policy, curriculum or procedures. Payment is usually in the form of compensation by the school as an hourly rate or portion of the CAP's FTE; in some cases, CAP's may choose to volunteer their time as community service.	• The CAP participates on school or district committees related to mental health topics (for example, on implementation of district-wide mental health screening; on the mental health impact of the school district's COVID-19 response, or a Special Education Advisory Committee) • The CAP supports schools and districts during times of school crisis (for example, after a school suicide or school shooting.) Examples of crisis response toolkits may be found at https://www.heardalliance.org/toolkit-intervention-crisis-response/, https://www.sprc.org/resources-programs/after-suicide-toolkit-schools & https://www.ready.gov/public-spaces • The CAP guides school district staff through planning, implementing and monitoring the development of Comprehensive School Mental Health Systems. The National Center for School Mental Health website (www.schoolmentalhealth.org) has a multitude of resources on this topic. • The CAP assists the school district in the planning and implementation of grant-funded mental health programs (such as the SAMHSA-funded Project AWARE state education grants https://www.samhsa.gov/grants/grant-announcements/sm-20-016)

DISCUSSION

This article sought to describe the evolution of different delivery models of school-based health and mental health, culminating in the current CSMHS initiative. The CMHS model offers an innovative approach to integrate mental health within school systems using a continuum ranging from prevention to intervention. By fostering positive school climate and universal social-emotional learning, this model helps to prevent the development of mental illness in some students. For those who develop early signs of distress, the model seeks to identify such students early through screening and mental health awareness. This focus on early identification and intervention potentially reduces the burden of full-blown mental illness. Finally, when students evidence significant mental health disorder, the model provides a continuum of services that meets the needs of the whole child and synchronizes school-based and community-based supports. For child and adolescent psychiatrists who are interested in system change, population health, prevention, health care equity, and integrated service delivery, these new developments in school-based mental health represent an exciting practice arena with a wealth of career opportunities that are likely to expand in the coming decade.

CLINICS CARE POINTS

- School-based health and mental health services have evolved over time into increasingly more integrated and comprehensive systems of service.
- Best practice in school-based mental health incorporates prevention, positive school climate, collaboration, social determinants of health, and public policy into a systems framework.
- Educators can be the eyes and ears and serve as expert consultants for the clinician, who can in turn be the expert consultant to help educators engage effectively with all students, especially those affected by severe anxiety, depression, and other mental health conditions.[39]
- Child and adolescent psychiatrists are uniquely positioned to provide direct service, consultation, and technical assistance to schools and school-based health centers on mental health.
- With suicide rates rising nationally, it is even more important to promote universal education about stress, distress, and disorders and how educators can participate in "upstream" primary prevention of serious complications from mental health conditions, including psychiatric hospitalization and suicide.
- By contributing to school-based mental health, child and adolescent psychiatrists can help to advance health equity.

DISCLOSURE

Dr. Ryst receives funding support from the Health Resources and Services Administration/Maternal and Child Health Bureau, the Nevada Division of Public and Behavioral Health and the Washoe County School District. Dr. Joshi is the co-editor of the forthcoming book: Thinking about Prescribing: The psychology of psychopharmacology with diverse youth and families. Washington, DC: APP, Inc 2021 (in press).

REFERENCES

1. Forness SR, Kim J, Walker HM. Prevalence of students with EBD: impact on general education. Beyond Behav 2012;21(2):3–10.
2. Langer DA, Wood JJ, Wood PA, et al. Mental health service use in schools and non-school-based outpatient settings: comparing predictors of service use. Sch Ment Health 2015;7:161–73.
3. Pescolido BA, Jensen PS, Martin JK, et al. Public knowledge and assessment of child mental health problems: findings from the National Stigma Study-Children. J Am Acad Child Adolesc Psychiatry 2008;47(3):339–49.

4. Searcey van Vulpen K, Habegar A, Simmons T. Rural school-based mental health services: parent perceptions of needs and barriers. Child Schools 2018;40(2): 104–11.
5. Doll B, Nastasi BK, Cornell L, et al. School-based mental health services: definitions and models of effective practice. J Appl Sch Psychol 2017;33(3):179–94.
6. Love HE, Schlitt J, Soleimanpour S, et al. Twenty years of school-based health care growth and expansion. Health Aff 2019;38(5):755–64.
7. North S, Dooley DG. School-based health care. Prim Care Clin 2020;47:231–40.
8. Arenson M, Hudson PJ, Lee NH, et al. The evidence on school-based health centers: a review. Glob Pediatr Health 2019;6:1–10.
9. Dunfee MN. School-based health centers in the United States: roots, reality and potential. J Sch Health 2020;90(8):665–70.
10. Love H, Soleimanpour S, Panchal N, et al. 2016-17 national school-based health center census report. On the School-Based Health Alliance website. Available at: https://www.sbh4all.org/wp-content/uploads/2019/05/2016-17-Census-Report-Final.pdf. Accessed February 17, 2021.
11. Hess RS, Pearrow M, Hazel CE, et al. Enhancing the behavioral and mental health services within school-based contexts. J Appl Sch Psychol 2017;33(3):214–32.
12. School health services. On CDC Healthy schools website. Available at: https://www.cdc.gov/healthyschools/schoolhealthservices.htm. Accessed February 17, 2021.
13. School-based health centers. On HRSA website. Available at: https://www.hrsa.gov/our-stories/school-health-centers/index.html. Accessed February 17, 2021.
14. Katz E. Realizing the potential of school-based health centers: a research brief and implementation guide. Available at: https://edredesign.org/files/edredesign/files/sbhc-brief-1?m=1601040943. Accessed February 17, 2021.
15. About school-based healthcare. On the School-Based Health Alliance website. Available at: https://www.sbh4all.org/school-health-care/aboutsbhcs/. Accessed February 17, 2021.
16. Rones M, Hoagwood K. School-based mental health services: a research review. Clin Child Fam Psychol Rev 2000;3:223–41.
17. Shelton AJ, Owens EW. Mental health services in the United States public high schools. J Sch Health 2021;91(1):70–6.
18. Foundations of school mental health. On the national center for school mental health website. Available at: http://www.schoolmentalhealth.org/Resources/Foundations-of-School-Mental-Health/. Accessed February 17, 2021.
19. Tiered framework. On the Center on PBIS website. Available at: https://www.pbis.org/pbis/tiered-framework. Accessed February 17, 2021.
20. Splett JW, Perales K, Halliday-Boykins CA, et al. Best practices for teaming and collaboration in the interconnected systems framework. J Appl Sch Psychol 2017; 33(4):347–68.
21. Lai K, Guo S, Ijadi-Maghsoodi R, et al. Bringing wellness to schools: opportunities for and challenges to mental health integration in school-based health centers. Psychiatr Serv 2016;67(12):1328–33.
22. Anglin TM, Naylor KE, Kaplan DW. Comprehensive school-based health care: high school students' use of medical, mental health and substance abuse services. Pediatrics 1996;97:318–30.
23. Larson S, Spetz J, Brindis CD, et al. Characteristic differences between school-based health centers with and without mental health providers: a review of national trends. J Pediatr Health Care 2017;31(4):484–92.

24. Knopf JA, Finnie RKC, Peng Y, et al. School-based health centers to advance health equity: a community guide systematic review. Am J Prev Med 2016; 51(1):114–26.
25. Gardiner T. Supporting health and educational outcomes through school-based health centers. Pediatr Nurs 2020;46(6):292–307.
26. Paschall MJ, Bersamin M. School-based health centers, depression and suicide risk among adolescents. Am J Prev Med 2018;54(1):44–50.
27. Robinson WL, Harper GW, Schoeny ME. Reducing substance use among African American adolescents: effectiveness of school-based health centers. Clin Psychol Sci Pract 2006;10(4):491–504.
28. Bains RM, Diallo AF. Mental health services in school-based health centers: systematic review. J Sch Nurs 2016;32(1):8–19.
29. Walker SC, Kerns SEU, Lyon AR, et al. Impact of school-based health center use on academic outcomes. J Adolesc Health 2010;46(3):251–7.
30. Kern L, Mathur SR, Albrecht SF, et al. The need for school-based mental health services and recommendations for implementation. Sch Ment Health 2017;9: 205–17.
31. Joshi SV, Ladegard K. Supporting SBHC students with mental health needs over the summer. Itasca (IL): AAP Council on School Health News; 2019.
32. Walter HJ, Kaye AJ, Dennery KM, et al. Three-year outcomes of a school-hospital partnership providing multitiered mental health services in urban schools. J Sch Health 2019;89(8):643–52.
33. Goddard A, Sullivan E, Fields P, et al. The future of telehealth in school-based health centers: lessons from COVID-19. J Pediatr Health Care 2020;00:1–6.
34. Adelman H, Taylor L. Embedding mental health ao schools change. 2021. Available at: http://omhp.psych.ucla.edu/barriersbook.pdf. Accessed February 27, 2021.
35. Beers N, Joshi SV. Increasing access to mental health services through reduction of stigma (invited commentary). Pediatrics 2020;145(6):e20200127.
36. Joshi SV, Jassim N. School-based interventions for mood disorders. In: Singh MK, editor. A clinical handbook for the diagnosis and treatment of pediatric onset mood disorders. Washington DC: Amer Psychiatric Assoc Press; 2019. p. 457–84.
37. Bostic JQ, Bagnell A. Psychiatric school consultation: an organizing framework and empowering techniques. Child Adolesc Psychiatr Clin N Am 2001; 10(1):1–12.
38. Joshi SV. School consultation and intervention. In: Steiner H, editor. Handbook of mental health interventions in children and adolescents: an integrated developmental approach. Hoboken, NJ: Jossey-Bass; 2004. p. 885–916.
39. Joshi SV, Jassim N, Mani N. Youth depression in school settings: assessment, interventions, and prevention. Child Adolesc Psychiatr Clin N Am 2019;28:349–62.

Engaging Pediatric Primary Care Clinicians in Collaborative and Integrated Care

Sourav Sengupta, MD, MPH[a,b]

KEYWORDS

- Collaborative • Integrated • Care • Pediatric • Primary • Engagement

KEY POINTS

- Pediatric primary care clinicians are being asked to manage an increasing breadth and depth of mental health challenges in the children and adolescents they treat.
- CAPs involved in CIC
  - need to develop excellent adult education capabilities to help PPCCs develop new pediatric behavioral knowledge and skills
  - provide timely consultations to clarify diagnosis, elucidate complex formulations, establish stepped treatment plans, and/or assist with appropriate service linkage or disposition challenges
  - generally provide brief, evidence-based treatment, bridging treatment, and assistance in urgent and crisis situations to pediatric patients and families directly in primary care practice
  - help PPCCs navigate regional mental health systems and advocate for sustainable payment structures supporting primary care mental health delivery

INTRODUCTION

Public health challenges connecting children and adolescents struggling with mental health issues with appropriate care are well known. Although 1 in 5 children are identified as struggling with mental health challenges, only 20% are able to access appropriate mental health services.[1–4] In this context, primary care clinicians are increasingly asked to manage complex emotional and behavioral challenges for children and adolescents in their practices, with an increasing proportion of ambulatory visits now involving a behavioral, emotional, or educational concern.[5] Pediatric primary care clinicians (PPCCs) generally report lacking the knowledge and skills to address these concerns in a busy primary care practice, compounding this complex

[a] Departments of Psychiatry & Pediatrics, Jacobs School of Medicine, University at Buffalo, Buffalo, NY, USA; [b] Children's Psychiatry Clinic of Oishei Children's Hospital, 1028 Main Street, Buffalo, NY 14202, USA
E-mail address: souravse@buffalo.edu

Child Adolesc Psychiatric Clin N Am 30 (2021) 767–776
https://doi.org/10.1016/j.chc.2021.07.003
1056-4993/21/© 2021 Elsevier Inc. All rights reserved.

public health challenge.[6] Child and adolescent psychiatrists (CAPs) must successfully engage PPCC partners in the effort to support children, adolescents, and families struggling with mental health challenges in our communities.

A broad spectrum of collaborative and integrated care (CIC) programs throughout the country works to build PPCCs' knowledge and skills in managing mild to moderate behavioral health issues, often while providing access to consultation and/or brief treatment.[7] These programs range from child psychiatry access programs (CPAPs) that allow PPCCs to call and consult with a CAP on challenging cases to primary care practices with colocated or integrated child therapists and CAPs to assist PPCCs on-site within their clinical workflow. Issues might range from learning how to guide a family struggling with their adolescent's self-injurious behavior to developing a stepped care model in the primary care practice for children struggling with anxiety. These are the kinds of supports that PPCCs need to be able to meet the needs of their patients with behavioral health challenges.

Not all PPCCs are prepared to engage in CIC practice. In general, PPCCs feel undertrained and inexperienced in delivering high-quality behavioral health care to their patients.[8] Beyond the appropriate knowledge and skills, addressing the increasingly complex emotional health needs of children, adolescents, and families within the context of a busy primary care practice requires an openness to change, a willingness to learn and develop new practices, and a will to encourage others within a practice to make the necessary transition. CAPs engaged in CIC must first assess a practice's readiness for change. Are there clinical and administrative champions that are interested in CIC? Are there healthy communication habits within the practice and with external collaborators? Can the practice dedicate time and personnel resources to establish and maintain CIC work? Is the practice prepared to meet regularly to assess and refine the CIC process and outcomes?[9,10] Although most practices will not be perfectly prepared to transition, having and further developing some of these attributes will help a practice transition to successful CIC work.

After assessing a practice's readiness for change, the CAP's ability to develop a working relationship with PPCCs and staff within a practice is key.[2] She or he may benefit by taking note of the practice's clinicians by name, how they like to practice, and the mental and behavioral health domains they do and do not need assistance with. She or he needs to understand how the front desk staff work, how medical assistants and nurses facilitate clinical care, and how practice managers decide upon and implement policy changes. Beyond being helpful with clinical issues that arise in daily practice, the CAP should be prepared to offer basic emotional support to all members of the practice team, from general questions about mental health to advice on how to help the team work through conflict. The CAP needs to be viewed by the primary care practice as knowledgeable, skilled, and available. To be able to help in meaningful ways requires good working relationships with the entire primary care team.

EDUCATION

Many CAPs involved in CIC help PPCCs build knowledge and skills in behavioral health management through some form of academic detailing.[11] Often scheduled during lunch or at preexisting practice meeting, these variably structured sessions generally focus on a key topic (eg, evidence-based treatments for depression in adolescents), often centered around epidemiology, assessment, interventions, case-based discussions, and/or an open period for questions.[12] These sessions are often didactic in nature, and learner participation can be relatively passive. Although the long-term retention of purely didactic educational sessions may be somewhat limited, these sessions can go a long way to normalize the importance of mental health care in the pediatric primary care setting. There are other models of targeted CIC education, including the case review session, in which an embedded CAP reviews predetermined or recently seen behavioral health cases with PPCCs. Generally, these strive to answer a specific clinical question, teach a general principle, and establish parameters for when and how to seek further assistance.

Several learning collaboratives have sought to imbue this model of brief educational interventions interspersed throughout a PPCC's busy schedule with an adult-learning model focused on practical, case-based learning. In some models, learners bring their own cases, presenting in a preestablished format to peer PPCCs as well as a multidisciplinary team of CAP, child mental health, and/or PPCC educators. The CAP and PPCC educators' roles are to facilitate an exploration of the case through peer questions, discussion, and suggestions. The group leaders mentor the group and facilitate the learning process, offering general principles and correcting factual inaccuracies, but are otherwise not the center of the learning process. In a series of such sessions, a learning collaborative can expose themselves to many different types and presentations of pediatric behavioral health issues, increase comfort in consulting with and advising peers, gain mastery in management of selected cases of interest, and develop lifelong learning habits that can help them address future behavioral health management issues as they arise.[11,13,14]

There are multiple examples of more intensive educational programming, in which CAPs, allied child mental health professionals, and/or PPCCs with extensive behavioral health training and expertise train PPCC learners to develop more in-depth pediatric mental health knowledge and skills.[11,15–18] Some more comprehensive programs combine one or more of the aforementioned approaches. PPCCs learn core skills and knowledge in an intensive training program and then go back to their practices and apply what they have learned with the ongoing support of a learning collaborative. Ongoing academic detailing (eg, "lunch and learns" or brief weekend workshops) serves to highlight more specific knowledge and skills (eg, engaging the traumatized child) or to briefly introduce core knowledge and skills to other practice team members who were unable to attend the more intensive training program.

To engage PPCCs in pediatric behavioral health care, CAPs involved in CIC need to develop excellent skills in adult education. A didactic session primarily focused on a slide presentation without opportunities for audience engagement, participation, and synthesis will often result in a passive learning process, with learners struggling to adopt critical knowledge and skills into daily practice. As with most educational interventions, it is critical for the CAP educator to focus on what she or he wishes the learners to know and be able to do by the end of the learning session. Working backward from these practical learning goals and objectives, the CAP educator ideally designs learning sessions that combine critical content with learning exercises designed to synthesize and apply the content. Educators often tend to attempt to cover too much content with insufficient opportunities to synthesize and apply what is being learned to promote retention and implementation into daily practice.[19]

In general, an hour-long session should have 2 to 3 interactive learning exercises to facilitate consolidation and synthesis of learning goals and objectives. For more basic skills, this could take the form of a group exercise, for example, grading a rating scale and creating a corresponding treatment plan. For more complex skills, for example, behavioral activation education, this could be accomplished by having participants pair off and practice with each other and then come back to reflect with the broader group. When experiential learning is a key component of the educational practice, the knowledge and skills reviewed in educational sessions can more easily be incorporated into future learning (eg, through a learning collaborative) or consultative work.

CONSULTATIONS

There are numerous models to clinically support PPCCs struggling with the management of specific clinical cases related to emotional or behavioral health challenges. The Substance Abuse and Mental Health Services Administration-Health Resources and Services Administration's Center for Integrated Health Solutions developed an integrated care framework laying out a 6-level spectrum of integration from no formal integration with only intermittent case discussion as needed to full-scale integration with shared electronic health records and treatment planning.[20] CAPs should be prepared to support PPCCs within the context of the integration framework that best fits a particular PPCC within his or her practice (**Fig. 1**).

Across the spectrum of integration, consultation can happen informally, as in the "curbside consult," when a PPCC verbally reviews a case or asks a clinical question from a CAP (who may or may not be directly involved in CIC). These are often more targeted questions, such as medication choice after an initial treatment failure, a diagnostic clarification, or navigation of a disposition challenge. CPAPs throughout the country offer more structured telephonic support.[2,11,13,17,18,21,22] A PPCC will call the CPAP to review a case with and receive guidance from a CAP that same day. CPAPs generally record basic information about the encounter so that if the PPCC calls again, the CAP will have some background information on which to base their subsequent advice. Some CPAPs send a brief communication to the calling PPCC shortly thereafter. In this form of telephonic or verbal consultation, a calm attitude of support and helpfulness is needed. The PPCC's busy clinical schedule must also be respected. A quick presentation of the problem, followed by appropriate clarifying questions, should then be followed by targeted clinical advice. Ideally, the CAP will also impart one or more general principles to guide the PPCC if a similar clinical scenario were to arise again. This is yet another opportunity to consolidate PPCC learning to help them build their pediatric mental health knowledge and skills.

Many CIC models and programs also provide a more formal clinical consultation, in which the PPCC will directly evaluate the patient and engage his or her family. A CAP's psychiatric evaluation can help to clarify diagnosis, elucidate a more complex formulation, establish a stepped treatment plan for the PPCC to follow, and/or assist with appropriate service linkage or disposition challenges. Formal consultations are ideal for cases in which the PPCC feels she or he can manage the case with further guidance from the CAP. As with other forms of consultation work, the subsequent case discussion and documentation serve to guide the ongoing treatment of an individual patient, as well as to clarify clinical decision-making and general principles in treating similar patients in the future.

Central to keeping PPCCs engaged in the CIC process is the ability to offer consultative support in a timely fashion. With waitlists for children and adolescents to see CAPs growing to weeks or months, the ability to consult a CAP in a timely fashion is critical to CIC work.[2] PPCCs can learn to rely on CAPs as reliable CIC partners if they can respond to informal "curbside" consultation requests within the same day. When creating clinical schedules for CIC-involved CAPs, it is important to reserve both time for consultations and time to coordinate with PPCCs, other mental health providers, schools, and other systems of care. For CAPs who are embedded within the primary care practice, it is important to be present in the shared clinical workspace. Documentation between patients should be completed in the same physical

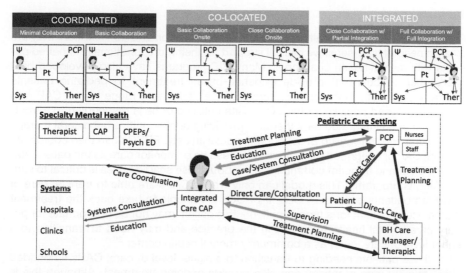

Fig. 1. CIC strategies for engaging pediatric primary care clinicians. CAPs involved in CIC engage primary care partners through consultation (blue), direct care (red), education (green), and treatment planning (purple). Depending on the level and type of integration, a CAP may be involved in a broad spectrum of these activities with the PPCC, integrated care therapist, specialty mental health providers, and the health care and other child-serving systems. BH, Behavioral Health; Sys, Systems; Ther, Therapist; PCP, Primary Care Practitioner; ED, Emergency Department; CPEP, Comprehensive Psychiatric Emergency Program; Pet, Specialty Mental Health.

space alongside PPCCs, allowing for increased access for informal consultation, ongoing care coordination for previously seen patients, and brief educational opportunities for PPCCs and staff.

Another important strategy to improve access to CAP consultation is telemedicine. The use of telemedicine platforms with appropriate privacy and audiovisual technology can facilitate a CAP being able to engage with patients and families across a broad geographic region, during times that are more convenient or accessible for the family or the CAP, and who might otherwise struggle to physically come in to the practice or another clinical location due to socioeconomic factors.[23] This format of engagement can also extend to reviewing relevant clinical cases after consultation with PPCCs.

It should be noted that there may be different philosophies and cultures relating to whether or not clinicians have their own children or family members treated within the practice setting at which they work. A PPCC or primary care practice staff might be used to bringing their own children or relatives into the practice for their pediatric health needs, whereas a CAP may be less likely to do so.[24,25] For a CAP engaged in CIC work, she or he may need to establish strategies for these scenarios beforehand. In these situations, it is important for the CAP to establish guidelines for appropriate privacy for the child and parent, adhere to preexisting guidelines regarding triaging and scheduling of cases based on clinical acuity, and maintain strict boundaries around family members' electronic health record access. Although it is important that the CAP make available the same consultative services to the children or family members of PPCC colleagues, she or he must also ensure that she or he does not allow the professional relationship to unduly influence the care or advice given to the patient and family.

TREATMENT

Although PPCCs are generally very receptive to education and consultation, they are often in need of time-sensitive clinical support for their more functionally impaired patients with mental health challenges. Many CIC programs have also developed brief intervention models that provide evidence-based treatment to pediatric patients and families directly in the primary care practice[7]; this might range from a CAP who sees a depressed adolescent for a few visits until she or he is responding to a treatment plan to an integrated care therapist providing brief cognitive behavioral therapy for a young child struggling at school with social anxiety. PPCCs can then coordinate with the CAP or integrated care therapist to resume or monitor care as the patient stabilizes. Clear and frequent communication about these shared cases is critical to successful CIC programs. This model can only work if CAPs are able to transfer care of stabilized patients back to PPCCs. If PPCCs are unable to take back the treatment of a particular patient (or a type of patient), this patient may not be appropriate for primary care mental health treatment in the practice and may need to transition to a higher level of care, such as a community mental health center.[26]

For these patients needing to transition to a higher level of care, CAPs embedded within primary care practices can also provide bridging treatment. Although this is generally preferable to a PPCC attempting to care for a patient with significant mental health needs that are more than the PPCC feels capable of handling, this treatment model generally requires more significant resources in terms of the CAP's clinical time available for direct care. Although this can provide improved mental health treatment of the patient and significant support to overstretched PPCCs, the CAP must be careful to maintain a sustainable balance of time available for new consultations, education, care coordination, as well as bridging treatment. Not infrequently, the CAP needs to assess the proportion of time dedicated to education, consultation, care coordination, and bridging treatment and adjust accordingly to allow for a sustainable allocation of clinical resources.

SYSTEM NAVIGATION

Although PPCCs are generally aware of clinically skilled specialist physicians to refer their patients to for complex medical challenges, they often struggle more with appropriate resource linkage and system navigation for their patients with complex mental health challenges. Partially, this may be due to differences in training and practice between PPCCs and child mental health clinicians, although stigma surrounding mental health issues in patients, families, and clinicians likely also plays a part.[27] Children, adolescents, and families with complex mental health challenges also often require more comprehensive psychosocial resources.[28] This may range from linkage with a quality outpatient therapist with expertise in trauma-informed care to positive parenting classes for new parents to an afterschool program with a social skills group. PPCCs and their staff work hard to understand what is available in their community and assemble resources they are able to share with families, but can feel at a loss guiding a family to the "best fit" or navigating systems when programs or practices are full.

CAPs involved in CIC need to have good working relationships with a regional network of outpatient therapists, community mental health centers, community service organizations, schools, psychiatric emergency programs, and inpatient psychiatric units. When CAPs are able to help PPCCs navigate the complex ecosystem of psychosocial services to determine what would be best for a particular child or adolescent, this may alleviate a significant clinical burden for PPCCs and may also help to assuage some of the emotional difficulties PPCCs may experience working with patients and families with more challenging behavioral health presentations.[29]

CRISIS MANAGEMENT

Perhaps no mental health scenario is more complex and taxing for PPCCs than an adolescent patient expressing acute suicidal ideation (SI). When SI is encountered in pediatric primary care, the approach is often to directly refer the patient and family to emergency medical services, the emergency department, or the psychiatric emergency program, if available in the region. Although a significant proportion of adolescents expressing SI will undoubtedly need emergent psychiatric evaluation, there is a broad spectrum of impairment associated with SI. Some patients and families will be receptive to education regarding depression, safety planning, and quickly engaging in mental health treatment. Other families may need education to differentiate nonsuicidal self-injurious behavior from suicidal ideation with active intent, plans, or acts of furtherance. And yet others will be in acute emotional distress and will, in fact, need to engage rapidly with emergency psychiatric services. CAPs involved in CIC cannot be an around-the-clock crisis service, yet must be prepared to help PPCC colleagues navigate mental health crises as they arise in the practice.[30] PPCCs can develop knowledge and skills to address mental health crises.[31,32] Triage nurses can be trained to improve screening skills, to follow preexisting treatment plans, or to direct families to the appropriate community mental health services rather than reflexively calling for emergency services. CAPs can consult with and guide PPCCs and their practices so that these situations, although always concerning, can feel more manageable.

ENGAGING HEALTH CARE SYSTEMS

Developing and implementing a CIC program inevitably requires a complex set of initial commitments, from finances to clinical services to administrative support. CAPs involved in CIC should be prepared to advocate alongside their PPCC colleagues with a broad spectrum of stakeholders to create and sustain CIC programs. This may involve making the value case for CIC, demonstrating the path toward cost-benefit or cost-effectiveness for a particular program within a particular health system, or planning how to meet the needs of a particularly complex set of patients (eg, children and adolescents with high-complexity medical and emotional health challenges). Regularly gathering feedback from PPCC colleagues, involving them in ongoing quality improvement processes, and shared advocacy are all important activities for the CAP involved in CIC.

Once a CIC program is developed and aiming for growth or expansion, the CAP may need to promote the program to inform regional PPCCs of the program's offerings. This promotion may take the form of brief or more extensive educational sessions for individual practices or regional pediatric groups. Engagement with other educational, public health, or community systems focused on children's welfare may also help in engaging new PPCCs.

CAPs should also be prepared to help PPCCs better understand how to ensure that they are appropriately compensated for mental health work done in the primary care setting, and this will require an understanding of current billing codes related to mental health care, documentation requirements, and local insurance payor practices regarding reimbursement. Similarly, CAPs should be prepared to implement billing strategies that reimburse for clinical work and care coordination work by the entire CIC team. Ultimately, this may involve advocating with regional insurance payors to not only adequately reimburse for direct clinical care by both PPCCs and CIC clinicians but also establish more comprehensive value-based reimbursement structures that acknowledge the downstream impacts of engaging children and adolescents earlier on in the course of their mental health challenges.[27,33]

SUMMARY

CAPs across the nation are increasingly involved in CIC work that builds the knowledge and skills of PPCCs to increasingly manage mild to moderate mental health challenges for children and adolescents in the primary care setting. CAPs need to develop their own set of diverse knowledge and skills to facilitate this process, from assessing a practice's readiness for change to engaging educational outreach to timely consultative guidance. PPCCs are being asked to manage an increasing breadth and depth of mental health challenges in the children and adolescents they treat. CAPs who can establish good working relationships, communicate clearly and efficiently, and facilitate the care of this population will be successful in engaging our PPCC partners in our shared goal of improving access to quality mental health treatment for children and adolescents in our communities.

CLINICS CARE POINTS

- PPCCs are being asked to manage an increasing breadth and depth of mental health challenges in the children and adolescents they treat.
- CAPs involved in CIC
  - need to develop excellent adult education capabilities to help PPCCs develop new pediatric behavioral knowledge and skills
  - provide timely consultations to clarify diagnosis, elucidate complex formulations, establish stepped treatment plans, and/or assist with appropriate service linkage or disposition challenges
  - generally provide brief, evidence-based treatment, bridging treatment, and assistance in urgent and crisis situations to pediatric patients and families directly in primary care practice
  - help PPCCs navigate regional mental health systems and advocate for sustainable payment structures supporting primary care mental health delivery.

DISCLOSURE

The author has nothing to disclose.

REFERENCES

1. Perou R, Bitsko RH, Blumberg SJ, et al. Mental health surveillance among children–United States, 2005-2011. MMWR Suppl 2013;62(2):1–35.
2. Martini RH, Hilt R, Marx L, et al. Best principles for integration of child psychiatry into the pediatric health home. Washington, DC: American Academy of Child and Adolescent Psychiatry; 2012.
3. Merikangas KR, He JP, Burstein M, et al. Lifetime prevalence of mental disorders in U.S. Adolescents: results from the national comorbidity survey replication–adolescent supplement (NCS-A). J Am Acad Child Adolesc Psychiatry 2010;49(10):980–9.
4. Merikangas KR, He JP, Brody D, et al. Prevalence and treatment of mental disorders among US children in the 2001-2004 NHANES. Pediatrics 2010;125(1):75–81.

5. Olfson M, Kroenke K, Wang S, et al. Trends in office-based mental health care provided by psychiatrists and primary care physicians. J Clin Psychiatry 2014; 75(3):247–53.
6. Horwitz SM, Storfer-Isser A, Kerker BD, et al. Barriers to the identification and management of psychosocial problems: changes from 2004 to 2013. Acad Pediatr 2015;15(6):613–20.
7. Asarnow JR, Rozenman M, Wiblin J, et al. Integrated medical-behavioral care compared with usual primary care for child and adolescent behavioral health: a meta-analysis. JAMA Pediatr 2015;169(10):929–37.
8. Fox HB, McManus MA, Klein JD, et al. Adolescent medicine training in pediatric residency programs. Pediatrics 2010;125(1):165–72.
9. Knox L, Brach C. The Practice Facilitation Handbook: Training Modules for New Facilitators and Their Trainers. Rockville, MD: Agency for Healthcare Research and Quality; June 2013. AHRQ Publication No. 13-0046-EF. p. 79-81.
10. King MA, Wissow LS, Baum RA. The role of organizational context in the implementation of a statewide initiative to integrate mental health services into pediatric primary care. Health Care Manage Rev 2018;43(3):206–17.
11. Kaye DL, Fornari V, Scharf M, et al. Description of a multi-university education and collaborative care child psychiatry access program: New York State's CAP PC. Gen Hosp Psychiatry 2017;48:32–6.
12. Soumerai SB, Avorn J. Principles of educational outreach ('academic detailing') to improve clinical decision making. JAMA 1990;263(4):549–56.
13. Gadomski AM, Wissow LS, Palinkas L, et al. Encouraging and sustaining integration of child mental health into primary care: interviews with primary care providers participating in Project TEACH (CAPES and CAP PC) in NY. Gen Hosp Psychiatry 2014;36(6):555–62.
14. McCaffrey ESN, Chang S, Farrelly G, et al. Mental health literacy in primary care: Canadian research and education for the advancement of child health (CanREACH). Evid Based Med 2017;22(4):123–31.
15. Wissow LS, Gadomski A, Roter D, et al. Improving child and parent mental health in primary care: a cluster-randomized trial of communication skills training. Pediatrics 2008;121(2):266–75.
16. Wissow L, Anthony B, Brown J, et al. A common factors approach to improving the mental health capacity of pediatric primary care. Adm Policy Ment Health 2008;35(4):305–18.
17. Walter HJ, Vernacchio L, Trudell EK, et al. Five-year outcomes of behavioral health integration in pediatric primary care. Pediatrics 2019;144(1):e20183243.
18. Hilt RJ, Romaire MA, McDonell MG, et al. The partnership access line: evaluating a child psychiatry consult program in Washington State. JAMA Pediatr 2013; 167(2):162–8.
19. Kaufman DM. Applying educational theory in practice. BMJ 2003;326(7382): 213–6.
20. Heath BWR P, Reynolds KA. A standard framework for levels of integrated healthcare. SAMHSA-HRSA Center for Integrated Health Solutions; 2013.
21. Sarvet B, Gold J, Bostic JQ, et al. Improving access to mental health care for children: the Massachusetts Child Psychiatry Access Project. Pediatrics 2010; 126(6):1191–200.
22. Straus JH, Sarvet B. Behavioral health care for children: the Massachusetts child psychiatry access project. Health Aff (Millwood) 2014;33(12):2153–61.
23. American Academy of Child and Adolescent Psychiatry (AACAP) Committee on Telepsychiatry and AACAP Committee on Quality Issues. Clinical update:

telepsychiatry with children and adolescents. J Am Acad Child Adolesc Psychiatry 2017;56(10):875–93.

24. Mattsson A, Derdeyn A. The child psychiatrist treating physicians' families. J Am Acad Child Psychiatry 1977;16(4):728–38.

25. Schneck SA. "Doctoring" doctors and their families. JAMA 1998;280(23): 2039–42.

26. McCue Horwitz S, Storfer-Isser A, Kerker BD, et al. Do on-site mental health professionals change pediatricians' responses to children's mental health problems? Acad Pediatr 2016;16(7):676–83.

27. American Academy of Child and Adolescent Psychiatry Committee on Health Care Access and Economics Task Force on Mental Health. Improving mental health services in primary care: reducing administrative and financial barriers to access and collaboration. Pediatrics 2009;123(4):1248–51.

28. Foy JM, Green CM, Earls MF, Committee On Psychosocial Aspects Of C, Family Health MHLWG. Mental health competencies for pediatric practice. Pediatrics 2019;144(5):e20192757.

29. Hine JF, Grennan AQ, Menousek KM, et al. Physician satisfaction with integrated behavioral health in pediatric primary care. J Prim Care Community Health 2017; 8(2):89–93.

30. Shain B, Committee On A. Suicide and suicide attempts in adolescents. Pediatrics 2016;138(1):e20161420.

31. Thompson EA, Eggert LL. Using the suicide risk screen to identify suicidal adolescents among potential high school dropouts. J Am Acad Child Adolesc Psychiatry 1999;38(12):1506–14.

32. Holi MM, Pelkonen M, Karlsson L, et al. Detecting suicidality among adolescent outpatients: evaluation of trained clinicians' suicidality assessment against a structured diagnostic assessment made by trained raters. BMC Psychiatry 2008;8:97.

33. Green CM, Foy JM, Earls MF, Committee On Psychosocial Aspects Of C, Family Health MHLWG. Achieving the pediatric mental health competencies. Pediatrics 2019;144(5):e20192758.

Rating Scales for Behavioral Health Screening System Within Pediatric Primary Care

Jessica K. Jeffrey, MD, MBA, MPH[a],*,
Angela L. Venegas-Murillo, MD, MPH[b,c], Rajeev Krishna, MD, PhD[d],
Nastassia J. Hajal, PhD[e]

KEYWORDS

- Behavioral health • Screening • Barriers to screening • Pediatric • Mental health
- Ratings scales • Rating scales validated in diverse samples

KEY POINTS

- Pediatric primary care professionals play a key role in identifying youth who would benefit from behavioral health services through universal screening.
- Many youth and families face barriers to accessing behavioral health screening, assessment, prevention, and treatment, including a lack of awareness of available resources, language barriers, stigma, and system mistrust.
- Child and adolescent psychiatrists may assist pediatric primary care practices with engaging youth and families around screening by assisting with identifying rating scales that have good psychometric characteristics across multiple languages, are validated in diverse samples, and are available within the public domain.
- Child and adolescent psychiatrists may partner with pediatric primary care professionals to assist with optimizing screening workflows and linkage to specialized behavioral health services.

[a] Department of Psychiatry & Biobehavioral Sciences, Division of Population Behavioral Health, Semel Institute for Neuroscience and Human Behavior, UCLA, 760 Westwood Plaza, A7-372A, Los Angeles, CA 90095, USA; [b] Department of Pediatrics, College of Medicine, Charles R. Drew University of Medicine & Science, 1748 East 118th Street, Room N147, Los Angeles, CA 90059, USA; [c] Department of General Internal Medicine and Health Service Research, UCLA Health, Los Angeles, CA, USA; [d] Behavioral Health, Department of Psychiatry, Nationwide Children's Hospital, 444 Butterfly Garden's Drive, Columbus, OH 43215, USA; [e] Department of Psychiatry & Biobehavioral Sciences, Division of Population Behavioral Health, UCLA-Semel Institute for Neuroscience and Human Behavior, 760 Westwood Plaza, A8-153, Los Angeles, CA 90095, USA
* Corresponding author.
E-mail address: JJeffrey@mednet.ucla.edu

Child Adolesc Psychiatric Clin N Am 30 (2021) 777–795
https://doi.org/10.1016/j.chc.2021.06.003
1056-4993/21/© 2021 The Authors. Published by Elsevier Inc. This is an open access article under the CC BY-NC-ND license (http://creativecommons.org/licenses/by-nc-nd/4.0/).

Abbreviations	
ACES	Adverse childhood experiences
PSC	Pediatric Symptom Checklist

INTRODUCTION

Within a given year, 13% to 20% of youth residing in the United States experience a behavioral health disorder.[1] Behavioral health conditions create significant morbidity. They negatively impact children and adolescents' developmental trajectory and are associated with impairment, such as lower academic achievement[2,3] and social dysfunction,[4,5] which may continue into adulthood. Many adults with behavioral health conditions report the onset of symptoms in childhood or adolescence. In fact, according to the World Health Organization, approximately 50% of behavioral health disorders begin by 14 years.[6] Notably, behavioral health challenges in childhood are also associated with physical illnesses in childhood and adulthood.[7,8]

On a societal level, behavioral health conditions are costly and those that persist into adulthood may be particularly so in terms of direct health care costs and lost productivity, especially when behavioral health conditions are comorbid with chronic medical conditions. Early intervention targeted to youth and families can mitigate the impact of behavioral health conditions and has been shown to result in favorable longer term economic outcomes, including increased earnings, tax revenue, and averted criminal justice costs.[9,10] The high prevalence, early onset, and immediate and long-term impacts of behavioral health conditions on youth and society[5] necessitates early identification of, and intervention for, these conditions. Yet, many youth and families face barriers to accessing behavioral health assessment, prevention, and treatment,[11,12] including a lack of awareness of available resources, language barriers, stigma, and system mistrust. For these families, pediatric primary care professionals can play a key role in identifying youth who would benefit from behavioral health services through universal screening, and subsequently linking families to behavioral health services in a way that feels connected to their overall health, and that is facilitated by a provider whom they already trust (the pediatric provider).

Although universal behavioral health screening in pediatric primary care is recommended by the American Academy of Pediatrics Task Force on Mental Health, the US Preventive Service Task Force, and required by Medicaid's Early and Periodic Screening, Diagnosis and Testing and commercial health plans through the Patient Protection and Affordable Care Act,[13] more than 50% of primary care professionals report never or rarely using a standardized behavioral health screening tool.[14] To be sure, there are barriers to conducting standardized behavioral health screening within busy pediatric primary care settings. These barriers include limited time and resources available for behavioral health screening, challenges with engaging youth and families around screening, and difficulties related to obtaining behavioral health consultation and treatment from specialists when indicated.[13,15] Child psychiatrists are well-positioned to guide pediatric primary care professionals on these important issues. This article reviews ways in which child psychiatrists can collaborate with pediatric primary care professionals to assist with adoption of behavioral health screening within pediatric primary care. Specifically, this article reviews the significance of adverse childhood experiences (ACEs) and discusses challenges related to screening for behavioral health conditions in diverse populations. Additionally, the article addresses considerations relating to workflows, introduces methods to optimize youth and family engagement, and provides a description of rating scales that may be used to screen for a wide variety of behavioral health conditions, with a focus on sociocultural considerations. A case study will illustrate the principles of screening for behavioral health conditions and will demonstrate collaboration between a child psychiatrist and pediatric primary care professionals to optimize treatment.

ADVERSE CHILDHOOD EXPERIENCES

Over the course of the past 2 decades, awareness of the connection between ACEs and chronic health conditions has become increasingly integrated into pediatric primary care. ACEs contribute significantly to the risk of developing many chronic illnesses in adulthood, such as diabetes, heart disease, and depression in a dose-dependent fashion, regardless of socioeconomic status.[16] Toxic stressors are experiences that frequently activate and increase the body's stress response system with each subsequent encounter leading to maladaptive coping mechanisms and impaired cognitive development.[17] Such toxic stressors include, but are not limited to, physical, verbal, and sexual abuse; witnessing intimate partner violence; family unit separation though divorce, incarceration, or immigration status; community violence; racism; discrimination; substance abuse; and exposure to mentally ill caregivers.[16,18-20] The effects of such toxic stressors, often viewed as traumatic life events, are amplified in the absence of a supportive adult relationship in a child's development.[17] The early impact of ACEs on children's development is demonstrated by increased behavioral health symptoms during childhood, including anxiety, depression, post-traumatic stress disorder, and externalizing or disruptive behavior. The burden of ACEs lies not only on the families affected but also on the communities in which they live.

Minority youth living in under-resourced communities are at increased risk of trauma exposure owing to existing structural inequities, including trauma related to immigration and contact with the immigration system, police brutality and justice system involvement, homelessness and housing instability, racism, gender identity discrimination, and community violence.[18,21-28] For example, more than 90% of low-income, African American youth reported exposure to more than 1 violent event in their lifetime, and slightly more than one-half have experienced someone close to them being shot or attacked.[28,29] In a low-income, predominately Latinx urban school district, 73% of sixth graders reported exposure to violence.[30] Another study found that two-thirds of adolescent immigrant Latinx youth had experienced a traumatic event.[31]

Yet, despite higher rates of trauma exposure and risk for poor mental health outcomes, under-resourced minority youth face significant inequities in receiving needed behavioral health resources.[32-34] In navigating the health care system, the idea of mistreatment in the clinical setting may deter youth and their families from participating in behavioral health services.[35] A recent study showed that Black youth experience racial discrimination on average about 5 times per day.[36] Another study showed that Black male youth were more likely to not seek behavioral health care owing to mistrust of service providers, shame, and stigma.[37] Among Latinx youth, migration trauma, acculturative stress, and discrimination is associated with lower levels of self-esteem and higher levels of depressive symptoms, anxiety, post-traumatic stress disorder, attention-deficit/hyperactivity disorder and conduct disorder.[38,39] Among immigrants, limited English proficiency and literacy limitations have also proven to be barriers in behavioral health screening among children.[38,40] The intersectionality of discrimination within behavioral health care is compounded with the experience of being overlooked in daily life, which makes it more difficult for people of color to seek help for deeper issues.[41] To build resilience, families need a supportive environment and guidance on how to overcome such experiences and their effects on overall well-being; pediatric primary care may be the ideal setting in which to achieve this.

The importance of screening and addressing adverse childhood events in the primary care setting has been well supported and advocated by the Centers for Disease Control and Prevention, the American Academy of Pediatrics, and various national health care groups in an effort to decrease the long-term health outcomes of such experiences. In the last 2 decades, many health care centers have adopted a trauma-informed care model, which is an organizational structure and treatment framework that involves understanding, recognizing, and responding to the effects of all types of trauma.[42] Through the work of California Surgeon General, Dr Nadine Burke Harris, ACEs Aware is a state-wide initiative to integrate ACEs screening into pediatric primary care practice, applying a trauma-informed care approach in discussing potential risk factors with families and providing linkages to social services and mental health care.[43] In addition, recent work raises the importance of structural inequalities in obtaining these resources; providers should be made aware of the need to engage in open discussion with their patients and caregivers on their lived experiences, potential barriers, and current strengths.[18]

Clinical Workflow

Child and adolescent psychiatrists may assist pediatric primary care practices with identifying workflows and psychometrically validated rating scales that will optimize behavioral health screening rates and increase the primary care professional's utility of screening. Considerations given to optimizing clinical workflows may decrease barriers associated with obtaining behavioral health screening in pediatric primary care practices. Pediatric primary care clinicians may be advised to initially administer a rating scale that will screen for a broad range of general behavioral health symptoms (internalizing and externalizing), with subsequent gating into rating scales that assess specific symptom domains for youth based on elevations on the initial broadband rating scale. The option to include gating minimizes the number of items asked, decreasing the overall time required to complete screening within busy practice settings.

Practically, clinical workflows are optimized when rating scales are brief, because this factor helps to prevent response fatigue, and thus facilitates obtaining more accurate information about symptoms.[44] Rating scales that are available within the public domain also increase ease of adoption, because this factor eliminates the financial and administrative burden required with purchasing rating scales.[44] Important considerations in screening include the rating scale availability in multiple languages and the option for oral administration of screening for caregivers. One study[40] showed that when Latinx families were screened with the Pediatric Symptom Checklist (PSC), there was a high rate of incomplete forms when the PSC was self-administered. However, completion rates improved when the PSC was delivered orally. Several factors may be at work, including potentially overcoming the inability to read and understand the terms on the written screener and greater confidence when answering verbally.

The administration of rating scales may be optimized when delivered electronically, because this practice assists with information capture, immediate availability of the data, and ease of scoring. Additionally, the documentation burden is decreased when the screening platform is integrated with an electronic medical record.[45] Importantly, for screeners to be a guide for pediatric primary care professionals' clinical interview and treatment plan, results must be available concurrent to the clinical encounter. Another important advantage of electronic screening is that youth prefer this modality to paper, because they believe this method is more likely to ensure confidentiality of responses.[46]

Optimizing Youth and Family Engagement and Providing Consultation

Youth and their caregivers may be more readily engaged around behavioral health screening when they understand the purpose of screening[44] and believe that screening will improve communication with their pediatric primary care professional and inform treatment options.[13] Child and adolescent psychiatrists may guide pediatric primary care professionals and their staff to introduce behavioral health rating scales as a way of universally, routinely, and confidentially assessing behavioral health vital signs. In fact, studies have reported that presenting behavioral health screening as universal and confidential increases rates of completion (85%–95%),[13] as compared with asking youth and families whether they would like to participate in screening (9%–45%).[47,48] Specifically, when administering behavioral health rating scales to youth, it is important to provide a private space to complete the rating scales and review with the youth who will have access to their answers and scores.

Child and adolescent psychiatrists can partner with pediatric primary care professionals to explore behavioral health screening results and engage families around the results. Child and adolescent psychiatrists can coach primary care professionals to review with youth the individual items they endorsed on the behavioral health screener and to discuss challenges in functioning they may be experiencing to further assess for the presence of a behavioral health disorder. Parental beliefs, attitudes, and availability play an important role in successful screening and engagement with behavioral health care for their children.[49,50] A discussion of the rating and interpretation of scale scores is an opportunity to provide psychoeducation, engage youth and caregivers in treatment, provide youth and caregivers with a sense of agency, and promote shared decision-making relating to treatment options.[44] Importantly, the screening itself may signal that these issues are appropriate for discussion during a primary care appointment and may prompt disclosure of behavioral health symptoms, even if not endorsed on the screen.[13] Within integrated care settings, the child psychiatrist may be consulted to support evaluation and initial treatment, as well as facilitate referral for specialty behavioral health care as needed.

RATING SCALE MEASURES

Providers may choose from a multitude of caregiver- and youth-report rating scales to measure youth behavioral health, as well as caregiver and family functioning. There are several factors to consider when selecting specific measures to be used in a clinical setting. First, rating scale measures should have strong psychometric properties.[51] Specifically, they must have adequate reliability (ie, items that make up each rating scale should assess the same construct and do so consistently) and validity (ie, the scale should measure the true underlying condition it was developed to assess). Many rating scales have established thresholds (or cutoff scores) for typical functioning that have been derived from normative data.[51] First, a measure is administered to a large sample of a specific population (eg, a community sample of preschool-aged boys in the United States); then, measure developers are able to determine particular scores indicative of functioning that is developmentally normative (typically below the 84th percentile of the entire sample), clinically elevated or high risk (between the 84th and 98th percentiles), and clinically significant (>98th percentile). The validity of these thresholds can subsequently be determined by evaluating their sensitivity and specificity (ability to correctly identify those with and without a specific clinical problem, respectively).[51] Rating scales with established thresholds are often most helpful for case conceptualization, treatment planning, ongoing outcome monitoring, and communication among health care professionals, because they provide an easy framework for understanding how a specific patient is functioning relevant to their peers.[52]

Importantly, in selecting rating scale measures to be used in clinical practice, it is critical to consider whether the measure's normative sample is representative of the patient population being served.[51] White, middle- and upper-middle class participants are overrepresented in many areas of psychological and psychiatric research, including in many psychometric and measure validation studies. In **Table 1**, we highlight several psychometrically sound, validated caregiver- and youth-report rating scales that may be helpful for pediatric primary care professionals, prioritizing measures that have been standardized on diverse samples and that are available in Spanish and other languages that are commonly spoken in North America. To facilitate adoption by pediatric professionals, we also prioritize measures that are freely available within the public domain.

Notably, there are several challenges in compiling a list of measures that share all of these characteristics (good psychometric characteristics across multiple languages, validated in diverse samples, and available within the public domain). Measures that have very large, nationally representative standardization samples, such as the Behavior Assessment System for Children[53] and the Achenbach System of Empirically-Based Assessment (ie, Child Behavior Checklist)[54] also tend to be those that incur cost. Although there is a continually growing body of work validating many public domain measures for a broad range of populations and in a variety of languages, there are some domains relevant to pediatric care in which public domain rating scale measures are unavailable or not yet validated. We include some of these measures where necessary (eg, the Parenting Stress Index).[55]

Within the public domain, we focus on measures whose standardization samples include diversity in terms of race, ethnicity, geographic region, and a variety of other demographic characteristics. In some cases, we include measures whose original normative samples were relatively homogenous, but that have since been validated more widely. In the same vein, we prioritized measures that are available in Spanish and other languages that are commonly spoken in North America. Even so, it is important to keep in mind that measures may function differently in different groups. For example, one study showed that the factor structure of a commonly used, nationally standardized measure of parent-reported preschooler functioning (Behavior Assessment System for Children-3 Behavioral and Emotional Screening System–Parent Preschool form) did not replicate for the Spanish-language form in a Latinx sample.[55] Thus, when using rating scales with patients who may not be represented in a measure's development or original normative sample, it is especially important to be aware of potential limitations of that measure and to use it in concert with other sources of clinical information and observation.

CASE STUDY*

Patient name and other identifying information have been altered to protect confidentiality.

Evelyn,* an 8-year-old Latinx girl, presented to clinic for her annual well-child visit. During the clinic visit, her pediatrician, Dr Venegas-Murillo, noticed that Evelyn had gained 20 pounds since her last visit and is now classified as obese. Her mother states that she offers her healthy food options and tries to limit fast food. Evelyn eats some

Table 1
Caregiver and youth rating scales

Measure	Form Information			Population Information					
					Normative Sample[b]				Psychometric Data Available from Other Racial, Ethnic, or Linguistic Groups?
	No. of Items[a]	Spanish Translation Available?	Other Translations Available?	n[c]	Child Ages (in Years)	Location	Clinical or Community Sample	Racial and Ethnic Breakdown	
General/Broadband Screening									
PSC[56]									
Patient report	17, 35	Y	Y	80,680	4–15	US	Community (pediatric practices)	Not reported	Y
Caregiver report	17, 35	Y	Y						
Anxiety symptoms									
Screen for Anxiety-Related Disorders[57]									
Patient report	41	Y	Y	190	9–19	US	Clinical (mood disorders clinic)	71.4% White; 22.8% African American; 5.8% Hispanic	Y
Caregiver report	41	Y	Y						
Spence[58–60]									
Patient report (8–12 y)	44	Y	Y	2052	8–12	Australia, the Netherlands	Community	Australian, Dutch	Y
Caregiver report (6–18 y)	38	Y	Y	484	6–18		Clinical/ community	Australian, Dutch	
Caregiver report (3–6 y)	34	Y	Y	1138	3–6		Community	Australian, Dutch	

(continued on next page)

Table 1
(continued)

| Measure | Form Information | | | Population Information | | | | | Psychometric Data Available from Other Racial, Ethnic, or Linguistic Groups? |
| | | | | Normative Sample[b] | | | | | |
	No. of Items[a]	Spanish Translation Available?	Other Translations Available?	n[c]	Child Ages (in Years)	Location	Clinical or Community Sample	Racial and Ethnic Breakdown	
Mood symptoms									
Mood and Feelings Questionnaire[c,d,61]									
Patient report	13, 33	Y	Y	172	6–17	US	Combined (28% clinical/psychiatric)	>75% White	Y
Caregiver report	13, 33	Y	Y						
PHQ-9[62]									
Patient report	9	Y	Y	442	13–17	US (Washington, Idaho)	Clinical	60% Female; 71% White; 10% Asian, 9.6% Black	
Childhood Severity of Psychiatric Illness[63]									
Caregiver/clinician report	34	Y	N	2666	M = 13 SD = 3.4	US (Illinois)	Participants were wards of Illinois Department of Child and Family Services	60% African American 32% White	
Preschool Feelings Checklist[64]									

Caregiver report	16	N	N	174	3–5.6	US (Washington)	Combined (23% clinical/psychiatric)	>85% White	Y

Attention problems

SNAP[65]

Caregiver report	90	Y	Y	1613	M = 8.4 SD = 1.6	US (Florida)	Community (school district)	70% White 30% African American	
Teacher report	90	Y	Y	1205	M = 7.7 SD = 1.8				

Vanderbilt[66]

Patient report	55	Y	Y	601	6–12	US (Oklahoma)	Community	57.4% White, 20.7% African American, 15% Hispanic, 4.2% Native American, 2.7% Other	
Caregiver report	43	Y	Y	587					

Disruptive behavior problems

Eyberg Child Behavior Inventory[67]

Caregiver report	36	Y	Y	798	2–16	US (Southeastern states)	Community	75% White, 19% African American, 3% Hispanic, 1% Asian, 1% Native American, 2% Mixed Ethnicity	Y

Affective Reactivity Index (irritability)[68]

(continued on next page)

Table 1
(continued)

Measure	Form Information			Population Information				
				Normative Sample[b]				
	No. of Items[a]	Spanish Translation Available?	Other Translations Available?	n[c]	Child Ages (in Years)	Location	Clinical or Community Sample[b]	Racial and Ethnic Breakdown	Psychometric Data Available from Other Racial, Ethnic, or Linguistic Groups?
Patient report	6	Y	Y	204	6–17 (M = 12.9, SD = 2.7)	US	Combined clinical and community	Not reported	Y
Caregiver report	6	Y	Y	194					
Traumatic stress symptoms									
Child and Adolescent Trauma Screen[69]									
Youth report (7–17 y)	15–40[a]	Y	Y	249	7–17	US (Washington and Oklahoma)	Clinical (outpatient clinics)	34.5% White, 14.1% African/ African American, 10% Hispanic, 5.2% Asian, 1.6% Pacific Islander, 1.2% American Native, 4% Other, 29.3% missing	Y
Caregiver report (7–17 y)	15–40[a]	Y	Y	267	7–17	US (Washington and Oklahoma)	Clinical (outpatient clinics)	38.2% White, 15.4% African/ African American, 9.7% Hispanic, 4.1% Asian, 1.9% Pacific Islander, 1.1% American Native, 1.9% Other, 27.7% missing	Y

Measure	Items			N	Age	Country	Setting	Race/Ethnicity	
Caregiver report (3–6 y)	15–40[a]	Y	Y	190	3–6	US (Washington and Oklahoma)	Clinical (outpatient clinics)	43.7% White, 14.2% African/African American, 7.4% Hispanic, 3.2% Asian, 2.6% Pacific Islander, .5% American Native, 3.2% Other, 25.3% missing	Y
Substance use									
CRAFFT[70]									
Patient report	6	Y	Y	538	14–18	US (Massachusetts)	Community (routine health care)	24.2% White, 50.6% African American, 18.8% Hispanic, 6.5% Asian or other	Y
Family screening									
Family Assessment Device[71]									
Caregiver and youth (12+) report	42	Y	Y	503	n/a	US	Mixed clinical and community	Not reported	Y
Parenting Stress Index [72]									
Caregiver self-report	36, 120	Y	Y	800	1 mo–12 y	US (Virginia)	Community (pediatric practices)	87% White, 10% African American, 3% Other	Y
Caregiver depressive symptoms: PHQ-9[73]									

(continued on next page)

Table 1
(continued)

| Measure | Form Information | | | | Population Information | | | | |
| | | | | | Normative Sample[b] | | | | Psychometric Data Available from Other Racial, Ethnic, or Linguistic Groups? |
	No. of Items[a]	Spanish Translation Available?	Other Translations Available?	n[c]	Child Ages (in Years)	Location	Clinical or Community Sample	Racial and Ethnic Breakdown	
Caregiver self-report	9	Y	Y	6000	n/a	US	Community (primary care and OB-GYN)	Sample 1: 79% White, 13% African American, 4% Hispanic Sample 2: 39% White, 15% African American, 39% Hispanic	Y
Caregiver support: Multidimensional Scale of Social Support[d,74]									
Caregiver self-report	12	Y	Y	275	n/a	US (North Carolina)	College students	Not reported	Y

Abbreviations: n/a, not applicable; PHQ, Patient Health Questionnaire.

[a] Number of items may vary based on gating, short vs long form, etc.

[b] Refers to sample upon which most current norms/cutoff scores were developed.

[c] For standardization samples that included countries outside of North America, numbers reflect only the subsample of North American participants).

[d] No suggested clinical cutoff scores.

vegetables but mostly eats carbohydrates like rice, bread, and tortillas; her favorite food is pizza. She does not drink much soda or juice. Evelyn gets most of her exercise at school; it is difficult for her to be active after school, because the family lives in a 2-bedroom apartment in an unsafe neighborhood. Notably, Evelyn's mother was recently diagnosed with type 2 diabetes; she reported understanding the importance of eating healthy but she too struggles with her weight. Evelyn's maternal grandmother also has type 2 diabetes.

The primary concern that Evelyn's mother expressed was related to Evelyn's academic performance, which had been on target up until this academic year. Her teachers have expressed concern that she is not performing well, and she may be held back a grade. Evelyn primarily struggles with reading and writing, and her family has difficulty supporting her with this; both parents are primarily Spanish-speaking, and Evelyn's 10-year-old brother gets impatient and argumentative when he is asked to help her. Evelyn has received tutoring for the past 3 months; it has helped a little but not enough to pass.

Behavioral Health Rating Scale Results

Mother report
- PSC: Within normal limits for all subscales
- Child and Adolescent Trauma Screen: 0 traumatic events endorsed
- Family Assessment Device: Elevated for unhealthy family functioning

Youth report
- PSC – Youth report: Clinically significant for Internalizing Problems and Total Symptom Score; Within normal limits for Externalizing Problems and Attention Problems
  - Other youth-report rating scales gated in owing to score on PSC Internalizing subscale
    - Screen for Child Anxiety Related Disorders: Clinically significant for generalized anxiety, separation anxiety, and school avoidance
    - Mood and Feelings Questionnaire: Clinically significant depressive symptoms
- Child and Adolescent Trauma Screen: 0 traumatic events endorsed

After a review of all of the information, Dr Venegas-Murillo considered the various possibilities for Evelyn's current health and development. Based on monitoring of weight over time, her mother's report of family medical history, and family's report of current eating and exercise routines, Evelyn's weight gain could be consistent with a biological predisposition to obesity (family history of obesity contributing to type 2 diabetes) and lack of developmentally appropriate, safe opportunities for exercise. The concern for recent decline in academic achievement (which did not significantly improve with tutoring) could be an entirely separate issue. It is not uncommon for learning disorders to go unnoticed until the mid-elementary years, when academic demands increase. However, before meeting with Evelyn and her mother, Dr Venegas-Murillo reviewed the results of the behavioral health rating scales that had been completed by Evelyn (using the English forms) and her mother (Spanish forms) while in the clinic waiting room. Both had completed the forms electronically, which allowed for immediate scoring so that Dr Venegas-Murillo could review the results before meeting with Evelyn and her mother. Evelyn's clinically significant scores on the youth report of the PSC, Screen for Child Anxiety Related Disorders, and Mood and Feeling Questionnaire suggested that she might be struggling with symptoms of an anxiety or mood disorder. Although neither Evelyn nor her mother reported Evelyn's having experienced the specific traumatic events listed on the Child and Adolescent Trauma Screen, Dr Venegas-Murillo noted Evelyn's mother's elevated score on the Family Assessment Device, suggesting some family-level stressors, as well as the report that their neighborhood was too unsafe for Evelyn to play outside after school. Importantly, anxiety and mood symptoms could be a cause for or a result of weight gain and academic problems—or both.

Dr Venegas-Murillo used the rating scale results to open up a conversation about Evelyn's behavioral health and their family's stress and well-being. She started by thanking them for taking the time to complete the questions about Evelyn's behavioral health vital signs and conveying how behavioral health is connected to physical health and well-being. When Evelyn's mother expressed surprise that Evelyn had reported mood and anxiety symptoms (which were not reflected in mother's report), Dr Venegas-Murillo explained that it is not uncommon for parents and children to have different reports on behavioral health rating scales—especially for internalizing symptoms like depression and anxiety. She also noted that Evelyn's mother's ratings on the Family Assessment Device suggested that their family might have had some challenges lately. Evelyn then turned to her mother, and with watery eyes, asked if she could share what had been going on. Her mother nodded, and Evelyn started to cry. In midst of tears, she told Dr Venegas-Murillo that her mother and father recently separated. They had been arguing frequently before the separation and she was worried about her mom's safety. She had been so consumed with anxiety that she had not been monitoring what she was eating. Mother started crying too, stating that she has a tendency to overeat when she is stressed and perhaps that was also happening for Evelyn. After assessing for safety, Dr Venegas-Murillo provided education to Evelyn and her mother about the relation between mood disorders and weight changes, noting that for many people, depressive symptoms lead to increased appetite and decreased motivation to engage in physical activity. Dr Venegas-Murillo also noted that mood and anxiety symptoms can have an impact on academic functioning; Evelyn admitted that sometimes she had a hard time paying attention at school because of her worry. Dr Venegas-Murillo recommended that, in addition to standard follow-up for weight gain (eg, ordered screening laboratory tests for diabetes, dyslipidemia, and metabolic disorders [thyroid dysfunction]; advised to increase physical activity and change diet), Evelyn receive an evaluation by a behavioral health provider who could further assess her behavioral health symptoms and recommend the appropriate type of therapy (eg, individual, family, or both), and whether an evaluation for psychiatric medication management would be appropriate. A behavioral health provider could also assist the family in requesting emotional support services at school, as well as an evaluation for learning difficulties, if appropriate. Finally, Dr Venegas-Murillo provided psychoeducation, brief practice, and informational handouts (Spanish and English) on healthy strategies for coping with stress, including diaphragmatic ("belly") breathing. To help facilitate follow-up with a behavioral health provider, Dr Venegas-Murillo calls the onsite behavioral health care provider and briefly introduces Evelyn and her mother to the provider before discharge, often referred as a warm handoff, to build rapport and trust.

SUMMARY

The high prevalence, early onset, and short- and long-term negative impact of behavioral health conditions necessitates early identification and treatment of behavioral health symptoms. Barriers to conducting standardized behavioral health screening within pediatric primary care settings include engaging youth and families around screening, limited time and resources available for this activity, and difficulties related to obtaining behavioral health consultation and treatment from specialists when indicated.[13,15] Child and adolescent psychiatrists may assist pediatric primary care practices with engaging youth and families around screening by assisting with identifying rating scales, with specific attention to measures that have good psychometric characteristics across multiple languages, are validated in diverse samples, and available within the public domain. Additionally, the child and adolescent psychiatrist may engage and partner with pediatric primary care professionals to assist with optimizing screening workflows and linkage to specialized behavioral health services, as needed.

CLINICS CARE POINTS

- Pediatric primary care professionals play a key role in identifying youth who would benefit from behavioral health services through universal screening.

- Many youth and families face barriers to accessing behavioral health screening, assessment, prevention, and treatment, including lack of awareness of available resources, language barriers, stigma, and system mistrust.

- Child and adolescent psychiatrists may assist pediatric primary care practices with engaging youth and families around screening by assisting with identifying rating scales that have good psychometric characteristics across multiple languages, are validated In diverse samples, and available within the public domain.

- Child and adolescent psychiatrists may partner with pediatric primary care professionals to assist with optimizing screening workflows and linkage to specialized behavioral health services.

DISCLOSURE

The authors have nothing to disclose.

REFERENCES

1. Perou R, Bitsko RH, Blumberg SJ, et al. Mental health surveillance among children–United States, 2005-2011. MMWR Suppl 2013;62(2):1–35.
2. Breslau J, Lane M, Sampson N, et al. Mental disorders and subsequent educational attainment in a US national sample. J Psychiatr Res 2008;42(9):708–16.
3. Murphy JM, Guzmán J, McCarthy AE, et al. Mental health predicts better academic outcomes: a longitudinal study of elementary school students in Chile. Child Psychiatry Hum Dev 2015;46(2):245–56.
4. Chen D, Drabick DAG, Burgers DE. A developmental perspective on peer rejection, deviant peer affiliation, and conduct problems among youth. Child Psychiatry Hum Dev 2015;46(6):823–38.
5. Tolan PH, Dodge KA. Children's mental health as a primary care and concern: a system for comprehensive support and service. Am Psychol 2005;60(6):601–14.
6. World Health Organization. Child and adolescent mental and brain health. Available at: https://www.who.int/activities/Improving-the-mental-and-brain-health-of-children-and-adolescents. Accessed February 26, 2021.

7. Goodwin RD, Sourander A, Duarte CS, et al. Do mental health problems in childhood predict chronic physical conditions among males in early adulthood? Evidence from a community-based prospective study. Psychol Med 2009;39(2): 301–11.

8. Vila G, Nollet-Clemençon C, Vera M, et al. Prevalence of DSM-IV disorders in children and adolescents with asthma versus diabetes. Can J Psychiatry Rev Can Psychiatr 1999;44(6):562–9.

9. Foster EM, Jones D, the Conduct Problems Prevention Research Group. Can a costly intervention be cost-effective?: an analysis of violence prevention. Arch Gen Psychiatry 2006;63(11):1284–91.

10. Reynolds AJ, Temple JA, White BAB, et al. Age 26 cost–benefit analysis of the child-parent center early education program. Child Dev 2011;82(1):379–404.

11. Kim G, Aguado Loi CX, Chiriboga DA, et al. Limited English proficiency as a barrier to mental health service use: a study of Latino and Asian immigrants with psychiatric disorders. J Psychiatr Res 2011;45(1):104–10.

12. Sentell T, Shumway M, Snowden L. Access to mental health treatment by English language proficiency and race/ethnicity. J Gen Intern Med 2007;22(2):289–93.

13. Wissow LS, Brown J, Fothergill KE, et al. Universal mental health screening in pediatric primary care: a systematic review. J Am Acad Child Adolesc Psychiatry 2013;52(11):1134–47.e23.

14. Kuhlthau K, Jellinek M, White G, et al. Increases in behavioral health screening in pediatric care for Massachusetts Medicaid patients. Arch Pediatr Adolesc Med 2011;165(7):660–4.

15. Beers LS, Godoy L, John T, et al. Mental health screening quality improvement learning collaborative in pediatric primary care. Pediatrics 2017;140(6). https://doi.org/10.1542/peds.2016-2966.

16. Felitti VJ, Anda RF, Nordenberg D, et al. Relationship of childhood abuse and household dysfunction to many of the leading causes of death in adults. The Adverse Childhood Experiences (ACE) study. [see comment]. Am J Prev Med 1998;14(4):245–58.

17. American Academy of Pediatrics. Discussion. Am J Prev Med 1998;14(4):361–4.

18. Bernard DL, Calhoun CD, Banks DE, et al. Making the "C-ACE" for a culturally-informed adverse childhood experiences framework to understand the pervasive mental health impact of racism on black youth. J Child Adolesc Trauma 2020. https://doi.org/10.1007/s40653-020-00319-9.

19. Bethell C, Gombojav N, Solloway M, et al. Adverse childhood experiences, resilience and mindfulness-based approaches: common denominator issues for children with emotional, mental, or behavioral problems. Child Adolesc Psychiatr Clin N Am 2016;25(2):139–56.

20. Cronholm PF, Forke CM, Wade R, et al. Adverse childhood experiences: expanding the concept of adversity. Am J Prev Med 2015;49(3):354–61.

21. Jackson DB, Fahmy C, Vaughn MG, et al. Police stops among at-risk youth: repercussions for mental health. J Adolesc Health 2019;65(5):627–32.

22. Gwadz MV, Nish D, Leonard NR, et al. Gender differences in traumatic events and rates of post-traumatic stress disorder among homeless youth. J Adolesc 2007;30(1):117–29.

23. Brunson RK, Miller J. Gender, race, and urban policing: the experience of African American youths. Gend Soc 2006;20(4):531–52.

24. de Arellano M, Andrews A, Reid-Quiñones K, et al. Immigration trauma among Hispanic youth: missed by trauma assessments and predictive of depression and PTSD symptoms. J Lat Psychol 2017;6. https://doi.org/10.1037/lat0000090.

25. López CM, Andrews AR III, Chisolm AM, et al. Racial/ethnic differences in trauma exposure and mental health disorders in adolescents. Cultur Divers Ethnic Minor Psychol 2017;23(3):382–7.

26. Merrick MT, Ford DC, Ports KA, et al. Prevalence of adverse childhood experiences from the 2011-2014 behavioral risk factor surveillance system in 23 states. JAMA Pediatr 2018;172(11):1038–44.

27. Yoshikawa H, Aber JL, Beardslee WR. The effects of poverty on the mental, emotional, and behavioral health of children and youth: implications for prevention. Am Psychol 2012;67(4):272–84.

28. Zona K, Milan S. Gender differences in the longitudinal impact of exposure to violence on mental health in urban youth. J Youth Adolesc 2011;40(12):1674–90.

29. Cooley-Strickland MR, Griffin RS, Darney D, et al. Urban African American youth exposed to community violence: a school-based anxiety preventive intervention efficacy study. J Prev Interv Community 2011;39(2):149–66.

30. Ramirez M, Wu Y, Kataoka S, et al. Youth violence across multiple dimensions: a study of violence, absenteeism, and suspensions among middle school children. J Pediatr 2012;161(3):542–6.e2.

31. Cleary SD, Snead R, Dietz-Chavez D, et al. Immigrant trauma and mental health outcomes among Latino youth. J Immigr Minor Health 2018;20(5):1053–9.

32. Alegria M, Vallas M, Pumariega AJ. Racial and ethnic disparities in pediatric mental health. Child Adolesc Psychiatr Clin N Am 2010;19(4):759–74.

33. Hough R, Hazen A, Soriano F, et al. Mental health care for Latinos: mental health services for Latino adolescents with psychiatric disorders. Psychiatr Serv Wash DC 2003;53:1556–62.

34. Olfson M, Druss BG, Marcus SC. Trends in mental health care among children and adolescents. N Engl J Med 2015;372(21):2029–38.

35. Fripp JA, Carlson RG. Exploring the influence of attitude and stigma on participation of African American and Latino populations in mental health services. J Multicult Couns Dev 2017;45(2):80–94.

36. English D, Lambert SF, Tynes BM, et al. Daily multidimensional racial discrimination among Black U.S. American adolescents. J Appl Dev Psychol 2020;66:101068.

37. Samuel IA. Utilization of mental health services among African-American male adolescents released from juvenile detention: examining reasons for within-group disparities in help-seeking behaviors. Child Adolesc Soc Work J 2015;32(1):33–43.

38. Caballero TM, DeCamp LR, Platt RE, et al. Addressing the mental health needs of Latino children in immigrant families. Clin Pediatr (Phila) 2017;56(7):648–58.

39. Ríos-Salas V, Larson A. Perceived discrimination, socioeconomic status, and mental health among Latino adolescents in US immigrant families. Child Youth Serv Rev 2015;56:116–25.

40. Hacker KA, Williams S, Myagmarjav E, et al. Persistence and change in pediatric symptom checklist scores over 10 to 18 months. Acad Pediatr 2009;9(4):270–7.

41. Cramer EP, Plummer S-B. People of color with disabilities: intersectionality as a framework for analyzing intimate partner violence in social, historical, and political contexts. J Aggress Maltreat Trauma 2009;18(2):162–81.

42. Hodas GR. Responding to childhood trauma: The promise and practice of trauma informed care. Abuse Services 2006;177:5–68.

43. Aware A. ACEs Aware master FAQ. Available at: https://www.acesaware.org/. Accessed February 26, 2021.

44. Jeffrey J, Klomhaus A, Enenbach M, et al. Self-report rating scales to guide measurement-based care in child and adolescent psychiatry. Child Adolesc Psychiatr Clin 2020;29(4):601–29.

45. Krishna R, Jeffrey J, Patel PD. Implementing measurement-based care in various practice settings. Child Adolesc Psychiatr Clin 2020;29(4):573–86.

46. Olson AL, Gaffney CA, Hedberg VA, et al. Use of inexpensive technology to enhance adolescent health screening and counseling. Arch Pediatr Adolesc Med 2009;163(2):172–7.

47. Horwitz SM, Hoagwood KE, Garner A, et al. No technological innovation is a panacea: a case series in quality improvement for primary care mental health services. Clin Pediatr (Phila) 2008;47(7):685–92.

48. Husky MM, Miller K, McGuire L, et al. Mental health screening of adolescents in pediatric practice. J Behav Health Serv Res 2011;38(2):159–69.

49. DosReis S, Barksdale CL, Sherman A, et al. Stigmatizing experiences of parents of children with a new diagnosis of ADHD. Psychiatr Serv Wash DC 2010;61(8): 811–6.

50. Pescosolido BA, Jensen PS, Martin JK, et al. Public knowledge and assessment of child mental health problems: findings from the National Stigma Study-Children. J Am Acad Child Adolesc Psychiatry 2008;47(3):339–49.

51. Myers K, Winters NC. Ten-year review of rating scales. I: overview of scale functioning, psychometric properties, and Selection. J Am Acad Child Adolesc Psychiatry 2002;41(2):114–22.

52. Sattler JM. Assessment of children: cognitive foundations. 5th edition. La Mesa (CA): Jerome M. Sattler, Publisher, Inc.; 2008.

53. Reynolds CR, Kamphaus RW. Behavior assessment system for children. 3rd edition. Pearson; 2015.

54. Achenbach TM. The Achenbach system of empirically based assessment (ASEBA): development, findings, theory, and applications. University of Vermont Research Center for Children, Youth, & Families; 2009.

55. Edyburn KL, Dowdy E, DiStefano C, et al. Measurement invariance of the English and Spanish BASC-3 behavioral and emotional screening system parent preschool forms. Early Child Res Q 2020;51:307–16.

56. Murphy JM, Bergmann P, Chiang C, et al. The PSC-17: subscale scores, reliability, and factor structure in a new national sample. Pediatrics 2016;138(3).

57. Birmaher B, Brent DA, Chiappetta L, et al. Psychometric properties of the screen for child anxiety related emotional disorders (SCARED): a replication study. J Am Acad Child Adolesc Psychiatry 1999;38(10):1230–6.

58. Spence SH, Rapee R, McDonald C, et al. The structure of anxiety symptoms among preschoolers. Behav Res Ther 2001;39(11):1293–316.

59. Spence SH. A measure of anxiety symptoms among children. Behav Res Ther 1998;36(5):545–66.

60. Nauta MH, Scholing A, Rapee RM, et al. A parent-report measure of children's anxiety: psychometric properties and comparison with child-report in a clinic and normal sample. Behav Res Ther 2004;42(7):813–39.

61. Angold AD, Stephen C. Development of a short questionnaire for use in epidemiological studies of depression in children and adolescents. Int Methods Psychiatr Res 1995;6(11):237–49.

62. Richardson LP, McCauley E, Grossman DC, et al. Evaluation of the patient health questionnaire-9 item for detecting major depression among adolescents. Pediatrics 2010;126(6):1117–23.

63. Leon SC, Uziel-Miller ND, Lyons JS, et al. Psychiatric hospital service utilization of children and adolescents in state custody. J Am Acad Child Adolesc Psychiatry 1999;38(3):305–10.

64. Luby JL, Heffelfinger A, Koenig-McNaught AL, et al. The Preschool Feelings checklist: a brief and sensitive screening measure for depression in young children. J Am Acad Child Adolesc Psychiatry 2004;43(6):708–17.

65. Bussing R, Fernandez M, Harwood M, et al. Parent and teacher SNAP-IV ratings of attention deficit hyperactivity disorder symptoms: psychometric properties and normative ratings from a school district sample. Assessment 2008;15(3):317–28.

66. Bard DE, Wolraich ML, Neas B, et al. The psychometric properties of the Vanderbilt attention-deficit hyperactivity disorder diagnostic parent rating scale in a community population. J Dev Behav Pediatr 2013;34(2):72–82.

67. Eyberg SM, Pincus DB. Eyberg child behavior inventory & Sutter-Eyberg student behavior inventory-revised: professional manual. Psychological Assessment Resources; 1999.

68. Stringaris A, Goodman R, Ferdinando S, et al. The Affective Reactivity Index: a concise irritability scale for clinical and research settings. J Child Psychol Psychiatry 2012;53(11):1109–17.

69. Sachser C, Berliner L, Holt T, et al. International development and psychometric properties of the child and adolescent trauma screen (CATS). J Affect Disord 2017;210:189–95.

70. Knight JR, Sherritt L, Shrier LA, et al. Validity of the CRAFFT substance abuse screening test among adolescent clinic patients. Arch Pediatr Adolesc Med 2002;156(6):607–14.

71. Miller IW, Ryan CE, Keitner GI, et al. The McMaster Approach to Families: theory, assessment, treatment and research. J Fam Ther 2000;22(2):168–89.

72. Abidin RR. Parenting stress index manual. 4th edition. Psychological Assessment Resources; 2012.

73. Kroenke K, Spitzer RL, Williams JBW. The PHQ-9. J Gen Intern Med 2001;16(9):606–13.

74. Zimet GD, Dahlem NW, Zimet SG, et al. The multidimensional scale of perceived social support. J Pers Assess 1988;52(1):30–41.

Collaboration Between Child and Adolescent Psychiatrists and Mental Health Pharmacists to Improve Treatment Outcomes

Debbie H. Lu, PharmD, MPH[a],*,
Julie A. Dopheide, PharmD, BCPP, FASHP[b], Dri Wang, PharmD, BCPP[c],
Jessica K. Jeffrey, MD, MPH, MBA, FAPA, DF-AACAP[d,e,f,g],
Steven Chen, PharmD, FASHP, FCSHP, FNAP[h]

KEYWORDS

- Child psychiatrist–pharmacist partnership
- Comprehensive medication management • Adverse drug events • Medication safety

KEY POINTS

- Medication safety in children and adolescents continues to be a public health concern.
- Interdisciplinary collaboration between child psychiatrists and pharmacists can improve health outcomes, including quality of care and patient safety.
- Pharmacists providing comprehensive medication management (CMM) can assist in the optimization of medication therapy.
- Racial disparities in psychotropic medication use are prevalent among youth. Pharmacist integration on the child psychiatry treatment team could help improve medication starts and persistence.

[a] Touro University California, College of Pharmacy, 1310 Club Drive, Vallejo, CA 94592, USA;
[b] Psychiatry and the Behavioral Sciences, University of Southern California School of Pharmacy and Keck School of Medicine, 1985 Zonal Avenue, Los Angeles, CA 90089, USA; [c] Otsuka Pharmaceutical Development and Comercialization, 508 Carnegie Center Drive, Princeton, New Jersey 08540, USA; [d] Division of Population Behavioral Health; [e] Division of Child and Adolescent Psychiatry; [f] UCLA Behavioral Health Associates; [g] UCLA Department of Psychiatry and Biobehavioral Sciences, UCLA Semel Institute of Neuroscience and Human Behavior, 760 Westwood Plaza, A7-372A, Los Angeles, CA 90024, USA; [h] Department of Clinical Pharmacy, University of Southern California School of Pharmacy, Los Angeles, CA 90089, USA
* Corresponding author.
E-mail address: debbiehlu99@hotmail.com

Child Adolesc Psychiatric Clin N Am 30 (2021) 797–808
https://doi.org/10.1016/j.chc.2021.06.006
1056-4993/21/© 2021 Elsevier Inc. All rights reserved.

childpsych.theclinics.com

Abbreviations	
CMM	comprehensive medication management
HEDIS	Healthcare Effectiveness Data and Information Set
ICS	inhaled corticosteroid
OIG	Office of the Inspector General
PGY1/2	Postgraduate Year One/Two (used only once but reverse-expanded for readers)
PharmD	Doctor of Pharmacy (Dorland's capitalizes professional titles; M-W Collegiate and M-W Medical do not)

INTRODUCTION

Despite increased federal funding for mental health care, access remains a long-standing challenge. Only 1 child psychiatrist is available for approximately every 10,000 children needing services in the United States.[1] High prevalence of mental health disorders and rising mental health diagnoses precipitated by the COVID-19 pandemic coupled with shortages of mental health professionals has led to further strain on an already fragile system.[2,3] Addressing the shortfall of mental health professionals requires an exploration of all untapped resources and identification of skilled professionals proven to deliver evidence-based services that optimize health outcomes. The clinical pharmacy, more commonly embedded with chronic disease treatment teams, is underutilized within the mental health space. Interdisciplinary collaboration between child psychiatrists and mental health pharmacists allows to have more time for patient evaluations and treatment sessions while a psychiatric pharmacist assists with valuable services such as therapeutic drug monitoring, medication care coordination for coexisting conditions, and medication education for family and care providers. This collaborative approach improves medication therapy outcomes, prevents adverse drug events, reduces the length of hospital stay, prevents emergency department visits, and improves patient and family treatment engagement and adherence.[4]

Many reports indicate that treatment with psychotropic medications among youth is often suboptimal, including major quality and safety concerns. In a 2015 study conducted by the Office of the Inspector General (OIG), board-certified child and adolescent psychiatrists conducted a peer evaluation of antipsychotic prescribing to youths in 5 states. Two-thirds of the 485 medical records reviewed demonstrated quality-of-care concerns, including poor monitoring (53%), treatment not appropriate (41%), too many medications (37%), treatment duration too long (34%), wrong dose (23%), patient too young for medication prescribed (17%), and treatment side effects that were unmanaged or mismanaged (7%).[5] In addition, child and adolescent psychiatrists and pediatricians prescribe up to 75% of all medications off-label,[6] further increasing the risk of medication-related harm.

Over the past 20 years, the unique sensitivities of children and adolescents to psychotropics, particularly antipsychotics and antidepressants, have been increasingly realized. An analysis of clinical trial data from pediatric and adult studies shows higher rates of sedation, weight gain, tachycardia, and agitation in youth given psychotropics compared with adults.[7] Youth are particularly prone to weight gain, dyslipidemia, and new-onset Type 2 diabetes from antipsychotics, with emerging evidence SSRIs may also increase Type 2 diabetes risk in youth.[8] Metformin is increasingly utilized as a strategy to prevent the development of metabolic side effects in youth prescribed psychotropics.[9] Yet despite a Food and Drug Administration warning[6] and OIG report on the need for metabolic syndrome monitoring when prescribing antipsychotic medications to children and adolescents, only a modest increase in glucose testing and lipid testing rates is evident. According to the National Committee for Quality Assurance, metabolic monitoring for children and adolescents on antipsychotics by commercial HMOs, commercial PPOs, and Medicaid HMOs for 2019 were 27.4%, 35.0%, and 37.8% compared with 2015 rates of 33.9%, 30.7%, and 29.8%, respectively.[10] Hyperprolactinemia is another psychotropic adverse effect requiring ongoing risk versus benefit assessment due to effects on sexual development and bone mass accrual. A 2-year study of 94 boys (mean age 11.8) treated with risperidone for aggression showed decreased trabecular bone mass and increased fracture risk.[11] The benefits of serotonergic antidepressants outweigh the risks for most youth with severe depression, OCD, or other evidence-based indications, but treatment-emergent hyperarousal and mood lability must be monitored carefully, and patient and family education on the risk of treatment-emergent suicidality is essential.[12] In addition to potential harm, these and other adverse drug effects may contribute to medication nonadherence if not appropriately managed.

In the United States, medication nonadherence is also influenced by health disparities, resulting in youth from ethnic minorities not consistently filling prescriptions for prescribed psychotropic medications. In a study using the 2004 to 2011 Medical Expenditure Panel Surveys, Cook and colleagues[13] found that Black and Latinx youths were significantly less likely to fill prescriptions for any psychotropic medication (5.0% and 3.4%, respectively) compared with 8.0% of Whites. Furthermore, the racial/ethnic differences persisted when assessing 3 subclasses of psychotropic medication (antidepressant, atypical antipsychotics, and stimulant) use. Pharmacist integration on the child psychiatry treatment team has been shown to improve medication starts and persistence through patient and family education and transitions of care programs that help address adverse effect management and treatment access.[4,14]

In this article, we will present the expanding role of clinical pharmacists in providing care for children and adolescents with psychiatric diagnoses. These diverse roles will be illustrated using case examples from a variety of care settings to provide child psychiatrists with context on how partnering with clinical pharmacists can improve treatment outcomes. We will share evidence and experience indicating which subpopulations would likely benefit most from a collaboration between child psychiatrists and clinical pharmacists and propose future initiatives to optimize child and adolescent mental health outcomes through psychiatrist-pharmacist partnerships.

THE ROLE OF PHARMACISTS IN OPTIMIZING MEDICATION THERAPY
Comprehensive Medication Management

Clinical pharmacists have demonstrated improved quality of care and lower costs for patients in a variety of settings, but particularly for the management of common chronic diseases such as diabetes, hypertension, dyslipidemia, and anticoagulation clinic.[15,16] Although medication nonadherence has been cited as the most common reason for treatment failure and incomplete attainment of clinical goals, data from 19 distinct medication management services found that inadequate pharmacotherapy (eg, subtherapeutic dosing or inadequate number of medications) and adverse drug effects make up more than 70% of the reasons for medication treatment failure.[17]

Clinical pharmacists today provide CMM to improve health outcomes, including patient safety and health care quality. "*Comprehensive medication management is defined as the standard of care that ensures each patient's medications (whether they are prescription, nonprescription, alternative, traditional, vitamins, or nutritional supplements) are individually assessed to determine that each medication is appropriate for the patient, effective for the medical condition, safe given the comorbidities and other medications being taken, and able to be taken by the patient as intended. Comprehensive medication management includes an individualized care plan that achieves the intended goals of therapy with appropriate follow-up to determine actual patient outcomes. This all occurs because the patient understands, agrees with, and actively participates in the treatment regimen, thus optimizing each patient's medication experience and clinical outcomes."*[18]

Through CMM, pharmacists play a critical role on the interdisciplinary team to ensure the optimization of medication therapy. For instance, during intake, the pharmacist commonly conducts a medical record review and provides an initial assessment of medication therapy to identify potentially significant drug interactions, suboptimal treatment of coexisting medical conditions, and evaluates laboratory test monitoring to verify the safety of a medication regimen. The clinical role for pharmacists on the team includes, but is not limited to, the following:

- Screen for drug interactions
- Advise on optimal/evidence-based dosing
- Compare clinically significant differences of formulations of medications
- Therapeutic drug monitoring
- Interpret and apply pharmacogenetic testing
- Ensure appropriate lab and rating scale monitoring
- Educate psychiatrists, patients, and their families about complementary therapeutics
- Educate family and caregivers on realistic expectations of medications
- Overcome Therapeutic Inertia, defined as when a patient is on several duplicate medications, and they are "finally" doing better (eg, the use of 2 antipsychotics with no enhanced clinical efficacy to the patient; rather, the combination is left on as a result of halted cross-titration). In these cases, the clinician/psychiatrist may hesitate to change any medication, leaving patients on medications that may not be necessary. A pharmacist can help identify which medication(s) can be safely and gradually tapered off to reduce side effects burden, costs, confusion, etc.
- Plan for rational deprescribing
- Coordinate care with other providers

Comprehensive Medication Management Practices

Recognizing the need to optimize psychotropic medication use, many states and counties have initiated programs to expand the role of pharmacists in psychiatric care (eg, the Alameda County and Los Angeles County Departments of Mental Health in California, Colorado Children's Hospital, Montana). Because psychotropic medications are often prescribed off-label for children with limited data and experience, state and county mental health departments and psychiatrists are increasingly partnering with pharmacists to improve medication therapy monitoring and the quality of care provided to youth with psychiatric diagnoses. Several states, including Texas,[12] Indiana,[19] and California[19] have published Pediatric Psychotropic Guidelines or Practice Parameters developed through collaborations between child psychiatrists and psychiatric pharmacists to elevate the quality of care for children and adolescents. Many states include child psychiatrists collaborating with pharmacists on Medicaid pharmacy and therapeutics committees and drug utilization review boards to improve medication safety.[20]

Although large scale trials measuring the impact of pharmacist interventions on mental health care outcomes are limited, many promising studies suggest psychiatric pharmacists managing medications for high-risk patients leads to better health and patient safety while lowering total health care costs. Tillman and colleagues[21] found pharmacy-driven transitional interventions within an adult inpatient psychiatric setting resulted in a nearly 50% reduction in 30-day hospital readmissions and ED presentations. Considering that nearly 20% of all readmissions nationwide occur within 30 days of discharge at a cost of approximately $52.4 billion, this is a critical area where pharmacists can add significant value and cost savings/avoidance. In another study, Cobb and colleagues evaluated the impact of psychiatric pharmacy CMM interventions in 154 patients receiving primary care services through a safety net clinic. More than half of the population had income below the Federal Poverty Level. Patients receiving psychiatric pharmacy CMM had an average of 10.1 medical and psychiatric conditions, 13.7 medications at baseline, and were complex in terms of medical/psychiatric conditions and medication therapy. The pharmacist identified an average of 5.6 medication-related problems per patient, with the most common psychiatric diagnoses as depression, insomnia, anxiety, and bipolar disorder. Actions taken by the pharmacist resulted in an estimated net cost savings of $90,484. The most common medication-related problems identified were adverse drug reactions, the use of unnecessary medications (eg, therapy duplication or no indication), unwarranted high doses of medications, and poor adherence.[22] CMM is starting to expand into the community pharmacy setting through programs such as the California Right Meds Collaborative (www.calrightmeds.org). In addition to the traditional services that psychiatrists are familiar with, highly accessible community pharmacists help improve medication-related safety and efficacy while providing local monitoring and surveillance for patients to reduce suicide risk.[23] These and other studies provide evidence that having psychiatric pharmacists manage medication therapy for complex patients in collaboration with psychiatrists is highly effective at achieving therapeutic outcomes of value to all stakeholders: patients, families, psychiatrists, and other team members, health systems, and payers.[4]

CASE 1—Educator Role (Inpatient and Outpatient Services)

A 14-year-old girl with a diagnosis of severe, single episode major depression presents to the clinic 1 week after release from the hospital following ingesting 10 aspirin tablets in a suicide attempt. She had been cutting intermittently over the past year and reported ongoing hopelessness and worthlessness. She has trouble concentrating and daily tearful episodes. She does not like online school and misses her friends. Her parents refused to sign her medication consent during her inpatient stay, stating, "We don't want our daughter to be addicted to drugs and we read about the increased risk of suicidality from antidepressants."

The psychiatric pharmacist plays an integral role in a child psychiatry practice by providing enhanced education for clients, caregivers, and family members regarding the effectiveness, safety, and necessary monitoring of psychiatric medications. The psychiatric pharmacist provided the following services for this patient:

1. As a supplement to education provided by the child psychiatrist, the psychiatric pharmacist met with the parents and caregivers to provide individual education on the safety and effectiveness of antidepressants in youth.
2. The psychiatric pharmacist met with the teen during hospitalization to engage her in a discussion of the benefits and side effects of antidepressant medication. During each education session, the psychiatric pharmacist emphasized the

importance of reporting all side effects and any changes in behavior (ie, aggression, mood swings, panic) after starting escitalopram 5 mg in the morning. The pharmacist emphasized changes in behavior could indicate the need for the child psychiatrist to assess for medication adjustment and suicide risk.

Medication educational groups are an added service that has been a part of child and adolescent psychiatry services for over 20 years. The benefits of these pharmacist-led groups on outcomes such as patient engagement are increasingly described in the literature.[24] Some child psychiatric treatment settings, including hospitals, day treatment centers, or clinics, offer weekly or monthly sessions for patients and family members. This type of group education can destigmatize taking medications, providing a forum for family engagement and much-needed support and monitoring. Psychiatric pharmacists provide a valuable role in improving outcomes for depression by encouraging proper administration, adherence, and monitoring.[14]

CASE 2—Evaluator Role—Comprehensive Medication Management (Outpatient Services)

A 10-year-old male with a past medical history of ADHD, autism spectrum disorder, oppositional defiant disorder, obsessive-compulsive disorder, chronic tics (eye blinking, shoulder shrugging), and asthma presents to the outpatient child psychiatry clinic with a chief complaint of worsening abnormal movements (tremor, shuffling walk) causing embarrassment in school. Blood pressure is 126/75, and heart rate is 105 beats/min. The child takes the following medications:

- Albuterol 90 mcg/actuation inhaler 2 puffs every 4 to 6 hours as needed for shortness of breath/wheezing
- Fluoxetine 40 mg by mouth daily
- Mixed amphetamine salts 20 mg daily
- Melatonin 3 mg by mouth every night at bedtime
- Polyethylene glycol 1 capful (17 g) by mouth daily
- Risperidone 3 mg by mouth daily

The psychiatric pharmacist identified several drug therapy issues to discuss with the child psychiatrist:

1. Screening for drug-drug interactions—fluoxetine inhibits CYP 2D6 and can decrease the metabolism of both risperidone and mixed amphetamine salts leading to a potential for increased side effects of both. Lowering the dose of risperidone to 1 mg daily compensates for the increased effect of risperidone due to the drug interaction with fluoxetine, further alleviating shuffling gait and tremor due to lower risperidone blood levels. The patient's aggression was controlled on the lower dose of risperidone.
2. Compare clinically significant differences in formulations of medications and preventing adverse effects—methylphenidate is a first-line stimulant for children because of overall better tolerability and similar effectiveness to mixed amphetamine salts.[9] It is less likely to worsen tics compared with amphetamine salts, and it is not a substrate for the CYP 2D6 enzyme.[25] The pharmacist assisted in obtaining collateral information on the reason for mixed amphetamine salts instead of methylphenidate. A switch from mixed amphetamine salts to methylphenidate removed the drug interaction contributing to the patient's elevated heart rate and tremor.

3. Coordinate care with other providers—This patient needed optimization of asthma management. Global Initiative for Asthma guidelines recommend, at minimum, daily inhaled corticosteroid (ICS) use or a symptom-driven combination of a long-acting beta2-adrenergic agonist with ICS rather than an as-needed albuterol inhaler.[26] Inhaled short-acting beta2-adrenergic agonists such as albuterol, particularly when overused, could contribute to tachycardia. The pharmacist coordinated asthma care with the patient's pediatrician, and the asthma regimen is optimized to inhaled fluticasone to minimize as-needed use of beta-adrenergic agonists.

CASE 3—Therapeutic Drug Monitoring and Pharmacogenomic Interpretation in a Case of Psychosis (Inpatient Services)

A 16-year-old male with a diagnosis of schizophrenia versus schizoaffective disorder has ongoing hallucinations, delusions, low mood, poor socialization, and cognitive impairment. The family recently moved from out of state for the mother's new job, and the family is here for an intake with a new child psychiatry team. History shows the patient had no improvement but did gain excessive weight from quetiapine 300 mg bid. The mother reports poor tolerability of aripiprazole due to restlessness. Over the past 2 months, the patient has taken risperidone 3 mg bid, benztropine 1 mg bid, and quetiapine 200 mg at bedtime (tapered from 600 mg/d). There has been no significant improvement in psychosis, but the patient is sleeping well. The patient gained 30 pounds since starting antipsychotic treatment at age 15, and the patient's BMI is now 32 kg/m². According to the mother and previous records, weight gain has been partially attenuated from adjunctive metformin 500 mg bid started 1 month ago. Current A1c is 5.6%, with lipid panel within normal limits. The child psychiatrist is considering a clozapine trial after checking to verify a therapeutic blood level of risperidone. The family also asks whether genetic testing could help find the right medicine.

This case illustrates several roles for the psychiatric pharmacist on the child psychiatry treatment team, including

1. Transition of care—patient recently relocated to the area. Medication history was obtained by the child psychiatry fellow, and the pharmacist verified the patient's medication utilization using prescription records from the pharmacy. Medication reconciliation is often a time-intensive process with many gaps in information; however, it is a crucial component of the transition-of-care process. An accurate medication history is important in preventing medication errors and allows for the assessment of a patient's current therapy to guide future treatment choices.

2. Therapeutic drug monitoring—the psychiatric pharmacist distributed a paper on therapeutic drug monitoring of antipsychotics[27] to the attending psychiatrist, child psychiatry fellows, and interdisciplinary students on the treatment team. Adequate trials of antipsychotics were verified through gathering collateral information and obtaining a blood level (48 ng/mL) of risperidone and 9-hydroxyrisperidone (or paliperidone). Renal function and metformin safety were verified.

3. Pharmacogenomic testing consult—pharmacogenomic tests can be beneficial for youth with known adverse effect sensitivities.[28] Based on the patient's current renal function, a pharmacogenomic test was deemed unnecessary prior to clozapine initiation as there was no reason to believe the patient would have an inability to metabolize clozapine based on past drug trials.[29] The patient was hospitalized during clozapine titration and discharged after a month of treatment and some improvement in psychosis and no further significant weight gain. Metformin was continued.

TARGETING YOUTH WITH MENTAL ILLNESS FOR COMPREHENSIVE MEDICATION MANAGEMENT

The case examples above illustrate how pharmacists can contribute to care optimization in a variety of psychiatric care settings. In particular, the cases demonstrate pharmacists' interventions in areas of enhanced medication education, evaluation of drug therapies, medication reconciliation during transitions of care, and optimizing the efficacy of drug therapy while minimizing risks for adverse effects. Of note, case #2 above illustrated the stigmatizing adverse effects of abnormal movements and tics resulting from drug interactions the pharmacist identified. The drug interactions identified and resolved by the pharmacist ended the needlessly prolonged suffering and embarrassment that the patient was experiencing, improving the patient's quality of life. Other high-value services that clinical pharmacists can provide include metabolic monitoring in conformance with HEDIS measures,[10] monitoring of narrow therapeutic index drugs, identifying high risk of misuse, and screening for dangerous drug interactions. Lastly, ensuring that patients, their families, and caregivers understand the purpose of their medications, how to use them appropriately, and how to self-monitor for adverse effects is vital to medication adherence. A lack of education regarding medications may lead to nonadherence and subsequent failure to reach treatment goals, increasing the risk for acute care utilization.

QUALIFICATIONS/CREDENTIALS FOR PHARMACISTS IN MENTAL HEALTH

As of 2004, all pharmacy programs in the United States have adopted the Doctor of Pharmacy (PharmD) degree, requiring student pharmacists to demonstrate doctorate level knowledge and skills in direct patient care prior to taking the pharmacist licensing examination. The PharmD curriculum is built over 3 to 4 years, similar to the duration of postgraduate training for student physicians.[30] In 2015, approximately 20% of pharmacy graduates pursued a PGY1 (Postgraduate Year One) residency.[31] The American Society of Health System Pharmacists, who manages the match program for pharmacy residencies in the United States, reported increased demand for and availability of residency training for pharmacy graduates. Between 2015 and 2020, the number of residency positions available increased 43% from 1861 to 2662. The number of PGY2 (Postgraduate Year Two) residency programs continues to grow, with 262 in ambulatory care, 95 in pediatrics, and 98 in psychiatric pharmacy as of 2020 along with several other specialty practice areas.[32] In addition to residency training, pharmacists can receive specialty certification. According to the Board of Pharmaceutical Specialties, 50,321 licensed pharmacists had active specialty certifications as of February 2021.[33] Board-certified pharmacists often practice in hospital, clinic, and community mental health settings where they can partner with child psychiatrists to improve quality of care for children and adolescents with psychiatric diagnoses.

THE INCREASING AVAILABILITY OF COMPREHENSIVE MEDICATION MANAGEMENT FOR MENTAL HEALTH PATIENTS: NEXT STEPS

The value of CMM for patients with mental health disorders has led to the successful integration of psychiatric pharmacists into a multitude of practice settings. Adding pharmacists to the care team has consistently demonstrated better health outcomes, medication safety, and satisfaction among patients and providers. However, because pharmacists are not recognized as health care providers under the Social Security Act, psychiatric pharmacy services cannot be billed for in the same manner as other providers; this is the primary rate-limiting factor preventing widespread availability of CMM services.

Several key strategies may help increase access to psychiatric pharmacy services. The first and most obvious is for pharmacists to receive national provider status, allowing payment for psychiatric pharmacy services. Because professional pharmacy societies have advocated for this for decades with limited success, pharmacist provider status is unlikely a near-term solution. The integration of clinical pharmacists into primary care teams has been more successful than in psychiatry, in large part due to evidence indicating that pharmacists are highly effective in improving pay for performance quality measures in primary care—eg, National Quality Forum measures and the Healthcare Effectiveness Data and Information Set (HEDIS). Value-based payment opportunities in psychiatry are currently limited; expanding these opportunities can help justify the addition of psychiatric pharmacists to the care team because most mental health conditions require optimal (safe and effective) medication therapy. This would also generate more scholarship evaluating the impact of psychiatric pharmacy services on measurable outcomes and aligns with the goals of contemporary thought leaders in child and adolescent psychiatry.[34] In addition, expanding collaboration between child psychiatrists and primary care providers could increase opportunities to network with primary care pharmacists offering CMM. Finally, most patients/lay public, physicians and other health care professionals, and senior health care leaders are unfamiliar with CMM services provided by psychiatric (and generally all) clinical pharmacists. A multidisciplinary public relations effort is needed, where physicians and senior health care leaders who understand and have benefited from psychiatric pharmacy services educate their peers about the value to patients, psychiatrists and members of the mental health team, and other key stakeholders.

DISCLOSURE

The authors reference unlabeled/unapproved/experimental and/or investigational (not FDA-approved) uses of drugs or products in this article.

D.H. Lu has nothing to disclose.

J.A. Dopheide has received honoraria as a consultant for Alkermes.

D. Wang is an employee of Otsuka Pharmaceutical. Otsuka Pharmaceutical neither endorses nor sponsors this publication.

S. Chen has nothing to disclose.

REFERENCES

1. McBain RK, Kofner A, Stein BD, et al. Growth and distribution of child psychiatrists in the United States: 2007–2016. Pediatrics 2019;144(6):e20191576.

2. Macdonald O, Smith K, Marven M, et al. How pharmacist prescribers can help meet the mental health consequences of COVID-19. Evid Based Ment Health 2020;23(4):131–2.

3. Panchal N, Kamal R, Cox C, et al. The implications of COVID-19 for mental health and substance use 2021. 2021. Available at: https://www.kff.org/coronavirus-covid-19/issue-brief/the-implications-of-covid-19-for-mental-health-and-substance-use/. Accessed February 25, 2021.

4. Werremeyer A, Bostwick J, Cobb C, et al. Impact of pharmacists on outcomes for patients with psychiatric or neurologic disorders. Ment Health Clin 2020;10(6):358–80.

5. Department of Health and Human Services Office of Inspector General. Second-generation antipsychotic drug use among medicaid-enrolled children: quality-of-care concerns. Available at: https://oig.hhs.gov/oei/reports/oei-07-12-00320.pdf. Accessed February 17, 2021.

6. Centers for Medicare & Medicaid Services. Atypical antipsychotic medications: use in pediatric patients. 2015. Available at: https://www.cms.gov/Medicare-Medicaid-Coordination/Fraud-Prevention/Medicaid-Integrity-Education/Pharmacy-Education-Materials/Downloads/atyp-antipsych-pediatric-factsheet11-14.pdf. Accessed February 25, 2021.

7. Liu XI, Schuette P, Burckart GJ, et al. A comparison of pediatric and adult safety studies for antipsychotic and antidepressant drugs submitted to the United States Food and drug administration. J Pediatr 2019;208:236–42.e3.

8. Sun JW, Hernández-Díaz S, Haneuse S, et al. Association of selective serotonin reuptake inhibitors with the risk of type 2 diabetes in children and adolescents. JAMA Psychiatry 2021;78(1):91.

9. Ellul P, Delorme R, Cortese S. Metformin for weight gain associated with second-Generation antipsychotics in children and adolescents: a systematic review and meta-analysis. CNS Drugs 2018;32(12):1103–12.

10. National Committee for Quality Assurance. Metabolic monitoring for children and adolescents on antipsychotics (APM). Available at: https://www.ncqa.org/hedis/measures/metabolic-monitoring-for-children-and-adolescents-on-antipsychotics/. Accessed February 21, 2021.

11. Calarge CA, Burns TL, Schlechte JA, et al. Longitudinal examination of the skeletal effects of selective serotonin reuptake inhibitors and risperidone in boys. J Clin Psychiatry 2015;76(05):607–13.

12. Texas Health and Human Services Commission. Psychotropic medication utilization Parameters for children and youth in behavioral health. Available at: https://hhs.texas.gov/sites/default/files/documents/doing-business-with-hhs/provider-portal/facilities-regulation/psychiatric/psychotropic-medication-utilization-parameters.pdf. Accessed December 28, 2020.

13. Cook BL, Carson NJ, Kafali EN, et al. Examining psychotropic medication use among youth in the U.S. by race/ethnicity and psychological impairment. Gen Hosp Psychiatry 2017;45:32–9.

14. Goldstone LW, DiPaula BA, Caballero J, et al. Improving medication-related outcomes for patients with psychiatric and neurologic disorders: value of psychiatric pharmacists as part of the health care team. Ment Health Clin 2015;5(1):1–28.

15. Margolis KL, Asche SE, Bergdall AR, et al. Effect of home blood pressure telemonitoring and pharmacist management on blood pressure control: a cluster randomized clinical trial. JAMA 2013;310(1):46.

16. Pellegrin KL, Krenk L, Oakes SJ, et al. Reductions in medication-related hospitalizations in older adults with medication management by hospital and community pharmacists: a quasi-experimental study. J Am Geriatr Soc 2017;65(1):212–9.

17. American College of Clinical Pharmacy. Comprehensive medication management in team-based care. Available at: https://www.pcpcc.org/sites/default/files/event-attachments/CMM%20Brief.pdf. Accessed February 1, 2021.

18. Patient-Centered Primary Care Collaborative (PCPCC). The patient-centered medical home: integrating comprehensive medication management to optimize patient outcomes resource guide. 2nd edition. Washington, DC: PCPCC; 2012. Available at: https://www.pcpcc.org/sites/default/files/media/medmanagement.pdf. Accessed February 17, 2021.

19. Los Angeles (California) department of mental health. Parameters 3.8 for use of psychotropic medication for children and adolescents. Available at: http://file.lacounty.gov/SDSInter/dmh/1071988_Paremeters3.8ForUseOfPsychotropicMedicationInChildrenAndAdolescents.pdf. Accessed February 20, 2021.

20. Medicaid medical directors learning network and rutgers center for education and research on mental health therapeutics. Antipsychotic medication use in Medicaid children and adolescents: report and resource guide from a 16-state study. Distributed by Rutgers CERTs at. Available at: http://rci.rutgers.edu/~cseap/MMDLNAPKIDS.html. Accessed February 20, 2021.

21. Tillman F, Greenberg J, Liu I, et al. Assessment of pharmacy-driven transitional interventions in hospitalized patients with psychiatric disorders. J Am Pharm Assoc 2020;60(1):22–30.

22. Cobb CD. Optimizing medication use with a pharmacist-provided comprehensive medication management service for patients with psychiatric disorders. Pharmacother J Hum Pharmacol Drug Ther 2014;34(12):1336–40.

23. Mospan CM, Gillette C, McKee J, et al. Community pharmacists as partners in reducing suicide risk. J Am Board Fam Med 2019;32(6):763–7.

24. James SM, Nahmias RA. Engaging hospitalized youth with medication education groups during the COVID-19 pandemic. Ment Health Clin 2020;10(5):305–6.

25. Dopheide J, Stutzman D, Pliszka S. Chapter 80: Attention deficit/hyperactivity disorder. In: DiPiro JT, Yee GC, Michael Posey L, et al, editors. Pharmacotherapy: a pathophysiologic approach, 11e. McGraw-Hill; 2019.

26. Global Initiative for Asthma. Global strategy for asthma management and prevention. 2020. Available at: https://ginasthma.org/wp-content/uploads/2020/06/GINA-2020-report_20_06_04-1-wms.pdf. Accessed February 15, 2021.

27. Schoretsanitis G, Kane JM, Correll CU, et al. Blood levels to optimize antipsychotic treatment in clinical practice: a joint consensus statement of the american society of clinical psychopharmacology and the therapeutic drug monitoring task force of the Arbeitsgemeinschaft für Neuropsychopharmakologie und Pharmakopsychiatrie. J Clin Psychiatry 2020;81(3):19cs13169.

28. U.S. Food and Drug Administration. The FDA Warns against the use of many genetic tests with unapproved claims to predict patient response to specific medications: FDA safety communication. 2018. Available at: https://www.fda.gov/medical-devices/safety-communications/fda-warns-against-use-many-genetic-tests-unapproved-claims-predict-patient-response-specific. Accessed December 20, 2020.

29. College of Psychiatric and Neurologic Pharmacists. Clozapine tool kit. Available at: https://cpnp.org/guideline/clozapine/2019. Accessed February 20, 2021.

30. Pollack S, Skillman S, Frogner B. Assessing the size and scope of the pharmacist workforce in the U.S. Center for health workforce studies. University of Washington; 2020. Available at: https://familymedicine.uw.edu/chws/publications/assessing-the-size-and-scope-of-the-pharmacist-workforce-in-the-us/. Accessed February 14, 2021.

31. Lyons K, Taylor DA, Minshew LM, et al. Student and school-level predictors of pharmacy residency attainment. Am J Pharm Educ 2018;82(2):6220.

32. American Society of Health-System Pharmacists. Resident matching program, summary of programs and positions offered and filled 2020 match - combined phase I and phase II. 2020. Available at: https://natmatch.com/ashprmp/stats/2020summpos.pdf. Accessed February 14, 2021.

33. Board of Pharmacy Specialties Website. Find a board certified pharmacist. 2020. Available at: https://www.bpsweb.org/find-a-board-certified-pharmacist. Accessed January 29, 2021.

34. Sarvet B, Jeffrey J, Grudnikoff E, et al. The time has come for measurement-based care in child and adolescent psychiatry. Child Adolesc Psychiatr Clin N Am 2020;29(4):xiii–xvi.

Child Psychiatrists and Psychologists
Enhanced Collaboration in Primary Care

Mark S. Borer, MD, DLFAPA, DLFAACAP[a,b],
Susan H. McDaniel, PhD, ABPP[c,d],*

KEYWORDS

- Integrated care • Collaborative care Model • Primary care behavioral health Model
- COVID-19 • Integrated care competencies • Practice transformation

KEY POINTS

- Increasing behavioral health integration into primary care increases access to child psychiatrists and psychologists.
- It is essential for child psychiatrists and psychologists to collaborate in integrated care systems.
- Mutual respect, and complementary skill sets and competencies, advance the effectiveness of care delivery in integrated care settings.

RESOURCES

Professional Associations with Involved Members and Resources about Integrated Primary Care:
- *Society of Clinical Child and Adolescent Psychology, Division 53 of the American Psychological Association*
- *https://sccap53.org.*
- *The Society for Developmental and Behavioral Pediatrics (SDBP). www.sdbp.org.*
- *Society of Pediatric Psychology www.societyofpediatricpsychology.org/ leadership. Division 54*

[a] Psychiatric Access for Central Delaware, P.A. Board Certified Child and Adolescent, General Adult Psychiatry; Family Psychiatry, 846 Walker Road Ste 32-2, Dover, DE 19904, USA; [b] Collaborative Psychiatry & Primary Care Consultation with Creatri(cs) Pro-Pack Toolkit®, Delaware Child Psychiatry Access Program (DCPAP) for Primary Care Professionals, Co-chair AACAP's Healthcare Access and Economics Committee; [c] Families & Health, Division of Collaborative Care and Wellness, Institute for the Family, Department of Psychiatry; [d] Department of Family Medicine, URMC Physician Communication Coaching Program, University of Rochester Medical Center, Rochester, NY, USA
* Corresponding author.SusanH2_McDaniel@URMC.Rochester.edu
E-mail address: SusanH2_McDaniel@URMC.Rochester.edu

Child Adolesc Psychiatric Clin N Am 30 (2021) 809–826
https://doi.org/10.1016/j.chc.2021.06.007
1056-4993/21/© 2021 Elsevier Inc. All rights reserved.

- *Society for Couple and Family Psychology—Division 43*
- *Collaborative Family Healthcare Association—an interdisciplinary association focused on integrated care. Some psychiatrists are members/on the board.*
- *American Academy of Child and Adolescent Psychiatry AACAP.org*
- *American Psychiatric Association APA.org*
- *American Academy of Pediatrics AAP.org*
- *American Academy of Family Physicians AAFP.org*

Educational and Training Resources:

PHQ-9 Patient Health Questionnaire https://www.ncbi.nlm.nih.gov/pmc/articles/PMC1495268/

GAD-7 Generalized Anxiety Disorder Questionnaire https://pubmed.ncbi.nlm.nih.gov/16717171/

CRAFFT (CAR, RELAX, ALONE, FORGET, FRIENDS, TROUBLE) https://crafft.org/get-the-crafft/

Training

- The annual 5-day interprofessional course each June at the University of Rochester Department of Psychiatry on Integrated Care and Medical Family Therapy (https://www.urmc.rochester.edu/psychiatry/institute-for-the-family/family-therapy/mfti.aspx).
- Nemours Children's Health System in Delaware offers an annual DREAMS conference (Developing and Researching Advanced Models of Integrated Primary Care, https://www.nemours.org/about/dream-ipc-conference.html).
- The Collaborative Family Healthcare Association annual meeting has Continuing Education focused on team-based integrated care.
- The American Psychiatric Association's (APA) 7-module, 2-part training course, developed in partnership with the AIMS Center, trains psychiatrists in Collaborative Care psychiatric consultation. It is free and earns continuing medical education credits.

KEY POINTS

- Increasing behavioral health integration into primary care increases access to child psychiatrists and psychologists.
- It is essential for child psychiatrists and psychologists to collaborate in integrated care systems.
- Mutual respect, and complementary skill sets and competencies, advance the effectiveness of care delivery in integrated care settings.

TERMS AND DEFINITIONS

"Child Psychiatrist" refers to "Child and Adolescent Psychiatrist"

"Psychologist" refers to doctoral-level child, family, pediatric, and health psychologists.

"Patients" versus "clients". "Patients" is the term used most in academic health centers and integrated care. "Clients" is the term more often used in independent practice and agencies. Because we both work primarily in health care, we use the term "patient" in this article, recognizing that either term must be defined based on partnership and respect.

"Integrated Care" refers to melding behavioral health, including psychology and child psychiatry, into "comprehensive primary care practices," "patient-centered medical homes" (PCMH), and networks. Child psychiatrists and psychologists may offer consulting or collaborative services, in person and increasingly by telehealth, or as "embedded" team members.

INTRODUCTION
The Roadmap

Many child psychiatrists collaborate routinely with psychologists; most develop collegial, mutually respectful relationships in optimizing care delivery.[1–6] This article presents ways in which our disciplines can and do collaborate with each other. Because of our important roles in reaching children and families in need, our focus is on our work together to integrate mental/behavioral health into primary care. We start with a description of our respective professions, their roles, and their training. We then describe the challenges both disciplines face as we consider the mental/behavioral health needs from a population health perspective. Far too frequently families are frustrated at their inability to find expedient access to a child psychiatrist or psychologist. Increasing access through primary care consultation and collaboration with mental health specialists, including those embedded in primary care practices, is a tremendous relief for those on long waiting lists, especially children being discharged from high-intensity care with no early follow-up scheduled. In addition, prescribing by primary care clinicians can preserve the child's ability to continue with their embedded psychologist or other behavioral health clinician.

We provide case examples of 2 integrated care models that begin to address these challenges: the University of Washington AIMS Center Collaborative Care Model (CoCM) and the Primary Care Behavioral Health Model (PCBH). Both are models in which child psychiatrists and psychologists can collaborate to support the Patient-Centered Medical Home (PCMH) in primary (and sometimes specialty) care. We describe how interprofessional teamwork can improve access and outcomes while invigorating our professions. We finish by providing a vision for the future of our collaboration.

The Premise

Together with our health professional colleagues, psychologists and child psychiatrists strive to promote a positive, health-oriented, collaborative approach to understanding and helping youth and families with an empathic approach attuned to the needs of the patient and family and sensitive to family culture.

As our disciplines transition from traditional or managed care delivery models to collaborative and integrated service models, this article's premise is that shared care delivery by child psychiatrists and psychologists results in optimal outcomes for youth. Data from Milliman show that delivery of mental health care is essential to both the physical and mental well-being of youth *and* their family members.[7,8] Patient outcomes and the patient/family experience ultimately determine the value of care. Teamwork between our professions, with primary care colleagues and with our patients/families, increases this value. As participants, leaders, innovators, even visionaries, together we enhance comprehensive primary care.

This premise in no way negates each discipline's strength on its own. Professional identity and skill development involve education and training in one's individual discipline as well as in concert with other professionals. Child and adolescent psychiatrists continue to resonate between the need to find common ground and further our professional collaborations with psychologists, and the need to identify, offer, and protect our own unique skills. As with other types of identity and brand development, we affirm ourselves not only with our individual training, skills, and perceptions, but also with the development and reflection of ourselves in relationships, including those professionals with whom we collaborate.

Our Identities and Training

Given the close collaboration between child psychiatrists and psychologists, what is different and what is similar about how we are trained and how we function? *A child and adolescent psychiatrist* is a physician with psychiatric training across the lifespan, as well as specialized training in youth development and their interactions with family, school, and community. Through study of both brain and mind, child psychiatrists bridge the medical, neurologic, developmental, dynamic, and interpersonal issues of youth. As of 2018, there were approximately 8300 practicing child and adolescent psychiatrists in the United States.[9] Shortages in this specialty cannot be resolved solely by opening up more training slots; it is imperative to increase patient access through collaboration with our partners, including psychologists.[10] It follows that connecting with our patients, directly and in collaboration with others, is an essential skill set.[11]

A practicing *psychologist* is a doctorally prepared health professional who has training in research methods and clinical techniques for the diagnosis and treatment of behavioral and mental health disorders. Psychologists work in health and mental health clinics, academic health centers, and independent practice, serving patients and families. They consult on and collaborate with other health professionals, including child psychiatrists and primary care clinicians, in the biopsychosocial care of patients with complex health problems. As of 2017, psychologists in clinical or counseling roles comprise approximately 51% of all psychologists, approximately 62,220, working in the United States (the other 49%, or 59,878, are research/academic psychologists). Twenty-three percent of all psychologists (approximately 28,060) are child-oriented practitioners.[12] The American Psychological Association (with 122,000 members) recognizes specialized training and Board recognition for specialties and subspecialty practices, including clinical, counseling, child, family, health, pediatric, school, neuro, and organizational psychology. All these practicing psychologists, with their various contexts and foci, are primed for collaboration with child psychiatrists.

Both child psychiatrists and psychologists may provide clinical interviewing, psychotherapy, program development and evaluation, systems assessment, leadership coaching, and team facilitation/effectiveness. Embedded psychologists also may act as leaders for on-site behavioral health teams.

To work together successfully, each discipline must understand its own competencies as well as those of the relevant team and its individuals. AACAP documents specific competencies for child psychiatrists.[13,14] McDaniel and colleagues[15] note specific competencies for psychologists in primary care. Common to both professions are complementary (not identical) skill sets in areas of science, systems leadership/administration, professionalism, relationships/interprofessionalism, practice management, and education/training. Unique roles for psychologists include advanced training in behavioral interventions, measurement, assessment, testing, program evaluation, and research.[15] Core functions of a psychiatrist include[3] the following capacities:

- *to perform difficult clinical evaluations*
- *to prescribe medications in complex situations*
- *to understand complex medical issues, and tolerate and manage acute crises*
- *to implement or support psychotherapies appropriate to youth and families[11]*

Table 1 provides a comparison of the education and training of our respective disciplines.

Traditionally, training in collaborative, interdisciplinary care is limited in our respective disciplines. It focuses primarily on securing one's individual professional identity rather than on in-depth learning about collaborative work with other professionals. Collaborative skill sets must begin with a collaborative attitude,[16] even passion, for working with other health professionals to provide comprehensive care that supports better outcomes for all patients, most especially those with complex problems requiring professionals with advanced degrees for assessment, consultation, and, at times, ongoing management.

Population Health and Mental Health

Understanding our individual and collaborative roles in promoting health and mental health requires an understanding of population health. In the past several decades, it has become increasingly clear that the US fee-for-service system focuses much more on treatment than prevention. This reality is especially the case for populations that do not have easy access to traditional health and mental health care services. The system does not result in the most effective or efficient care for the most people. For these reasons, and the need to contain sky-rocketing health care costs, population health approaches have developed for a minority in the United States and for many globally.

The population health pyramid in **Figure 1**[17] describes 3 levels of service needed for physical and mental/behavioral health care. The bottom and largest level is Universal: for all children and families. This level focuses on education, prevention, and general support, for issues such as nutrition, exercise, stress, conflict management, sexual health, and substance use. Organized modalities at this level include medical visits for well-child care, behavioral health screening, parent training, and psychoeducation.

The second level is considerably smaller, and targets children and families with risk factors who are in acute distress. Approximately 75% of children and adolescents with psychiatric disorders are seen in their pediatrician's office, leading the American Academy of Pediatrics (AAP) to advocate for behavioral health integration. This level of care is given often by members of the primary care team and/or by master's-level behavioral health clinicians who provide extra support, anticipatory guidance, and brief intervention while monitoring for ongoing distress. Examples at this level include parent groups, and psychotropic medication and psychotherapy groups for mildly depressed or anxious adolescents. Many family medicine residencies provide integrated training for their clinicians, and fairly extensive training in psychosocial

Table 1	
Education and training of child psychiatrists and practicing psychologists	
Child and Adolescent Psychiatrist	**Practicing Psychologist**
Medical school: 4 y	Graduate school: 4–6 y
Medical internship and residency: 3–4 y[a]	Internship: 1 y
Fellowship: 2 y	Fellowship: 1–2 y[b]
Total = 9 y	Total = 6–9 y

[a] The first year of a child fellowship may occur during the fourth year of residency.
[b] Optional but frequent for practicing psychologists focused on integrated care.

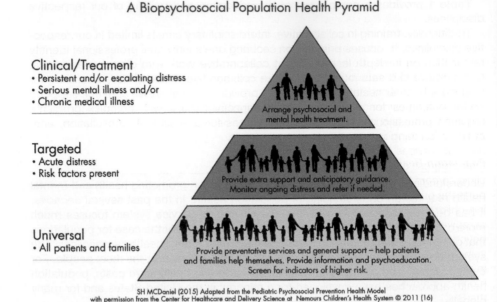

Fig. 1. A biosocial population health pyramid.[17]

medicine. They continue to seek training on youth mental health issues from child psychiatrists and psychologists.[17,18]

The top of the pyramid involves the smallest number of children or adults, that is, those with persistent and/or escalating distress, and/or serious medical or mental illness. This level requires clinical consultation and care by professionals with the most training, including child psychiatrists and psychologists. These patients are the most likely to be referred for tertiary medical or mental health care.

The more we focus on a population health approach, the greater the importance of a collaborative, interprofessional leadership team at the center. This leadership team then supports the wider teams providing comprehensive care, including primary care, schools, and community agencies.

Collaborative and Integrated Care

The need, skills, and process of interprofessional teamwork

The inadequate numbers of trained mental health professionals in our workforce to meet the needs of our population at Levels 2 and 3 in the population health pyramid make collaboration critically important between child psychiatrists and psychologists, along with other mental health and substance abuse professionals. The National Council on Behavioral Health Medical Director Institute stated: *Solutions [to access] cannot rely on a single change in the field such as recruiting more psychiatrists or raising payment.... Rather, the solutions depend on a combination of interrelated fields that require support from a range of stakeholders.*[19] This situation is most acute when attempting to access child and adolescent psychiatric services. This is why we must support, by training, collaborative skill-building, and by incentives that include decreased hassles and reasonable compensation, the presence of child psychiatrists and psychologists, for some portion of their practice, in the contact with, training of, and service to, primary care professional teams and their patients.

We describe as follows 2 of the major collaborative delivery models that seek to meet these needs: the University of Washington CoCM, and the PCBH. Both models value the role of the child psychiatrist and psychologist, whether care is delivered in direct relationship with the patient or indirectly through professional collaboration and communication. Both approaches seek to improve the welfare of the patient and family, who remain both the focus of care, and essential partners in contributing to and implementing that care.

CoCM is an evidence-based model, initially developed for adults with serious and chronic mental and medical illness,[20] currently being used with children and adolescents.[21,22] The model emphasizes the use of screening tools to identify patients in need of services. Patients who screen positive are enrolled in a program that tracks their progress over time. The program uses a child psychiatrist and a behavioral health clinician/care manager (BHC). The child psychiatrist serves as a consultant who supports the primary care physician and the BHC (often a nurse or social worker) in treating children with mental/behavioral health problems in concert with their parents/caregivers. Typically, these clinical presentations have been refractory to care or beyond the experience of the primary care team. The psychiatrist conducts weekly review sessions with the BHC, focusing on patients who are having difficulty progressing in their treatment. The psychiatrist directly evaluates the patient when needed, but more commonly provides recommendations to either the primary care clinician or the BHC (**Fig. 2**).

Psychologists can be important contributors in this model, whether providing care as embedded in the integrated practice, or through referral to outside practices. Their services may also include testing, measurement/rating scale consultant, team facilitator, or leadership coach.

The following is a case example of the CoCM in which the collaborative relationship with a privately practicing child psychiatrist formed the basis for a subsequent relationship for this primary care practice with the state's primary care access program.

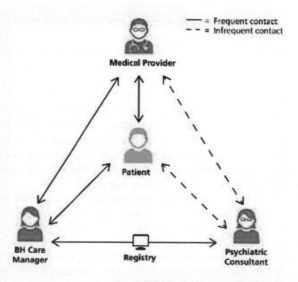

Fig. 2. The collaborative care team model. (Used with permission from the University of Washington AIMS Center, 6/10/2021.)

This program created additional access to collaboration with a child psychiatrist, while the practice also worked to embed a psychologist as another step toward integration.

In a rural primary care practice, Dr Pediatrician sought help in caring for Johnny, a male patient, age 17, who was abusing marijuana and recently "totaled his car" while high. Johnny was anxious and depressed, with a family history of bipolar disorder. He was showing intermittent agitation and verbal aggression. He was working with Dr Psychologist who was treating his anxiety and depression with cognitive behavioral therapy (CBT). The pediatric practice had Ms SW, a licensed clinical social worker, who was the practice's BHC collaborating and reinforcing the psychologist's recommended interventions. Johnny's parents were understandably distressed. Their solution to the car accident and drug use was to ground Johnny; they were not sure how else to handle his marijuana use. Ms SW sought consultation on behalf of Dr Pediatrician from Dr Child Psychiatrist to discuss strategies to help Johnny in particular, and teens abusing marijuana in general.

Diagnostic considerations: substance use disorder (SUD), anxiety, depression, rule out bipolar disorder
Dr Child Psychiatrist and Ms SW discussed considerations for care and further treatment planning. Ms SW then discussed treatment planning and prescribing with Dr Pediatrician, as follows:

1. *Due to daily smoking and defiance of parental rules, along with a recent motor vehicle accident (MVA), consider referral to an addictions outpatient program for additional assessment and therapeutic support. Parents should manage the car keys. Offer incentives for Johnny to go for the assessment, and age-appropriate consequences if he initially refuses to attend.*
2. *Screening tools: A substance abuse screener such as the CRAFFT (CAR, RELAX, ALONE, FORGET, FRIENDS, TROUBLE) to document and measure improvements[23] — or setbacks necessitating a higher intensity of services, PHQ-9 (Pediatric Health Questionnaire) for depression and suicidal ideation, GAD-7 (Generalized Anxiety Disorder Questionnaire) for anxiety. (Dr Child Psychiatrist, Dr Psychologist, and Ms SW will then select those measures to be entered and reviewed weekly on the practice registry.)*
3. *Assessment of any suicidal ideation or intent contributing to the MVA.*
4. *Intermittent urine drug screens are important to support motivation and monitoring.*
5. *Inform parents of crisis services available through Child Priority Response. His insurer may also have an online care manager for phone support.*
6. *Continue Dr Psychologist–instituted and monitored CBT, as well as any additional individual and family psychotherapy for anxiety and depression that can be helpful to reduce symptoms and promote abstinence. (As a result of Dr Psychologist's work with this teen and family, as well as others, the primary care practice began discussing embedding him for 2 d/wk at this point).*
7. *Discuss the marijuana use with Dr Psychologist for multidisciplinary treatment planning, as interspecialty input and collaboration leads to best outcomes. Medication and therapy for underlying mood, anxiety, and anger will enhance Johnny's potential benefit from addictions treatment.*
8. *Talk to patient and parents about finding a confidante and a small fellowship group of people who do not abuse substances. This can supplement available 12 step programs, including Zoom 12 Step, which increases access.*
9. *If parents use substances, encourage them to hold off or get help themselves to model abstinence for their son.*

10. *A second generation antipsychotic or valproate extended release may help with the mood and anger symptoms, and may be less likely to aggravate mood swings than a selective serotonin reuptake inhibitor (SSRI) due to bipolar disorder in his family history.*
11. *Once stabilized on medication and able to reduce or refrain from marijuana use, this teen is more likely to adhere to treatment and apply himself to academics and post–high school plans.*
12. *Suggest monitoring for signs of marijuana withdrawal over the next month as a possible contributor to his anxiety or moodiness.*
13. *Recommend the pediatrician manage psychiatric medications, with follow-up access to the child psychiatrist as needed. If treatment is refractory, referral to child psychiatry services may be needed in light of multiple diagnostic and therapeutic issues.*

It is noteworthy that the child psychiatrist, a private practitioner, received an invitation for ongoing collaboration with this pediatric practice following the psychiatrist's presentation on collaborative care at a statewide pediatric conference. This arrangement has led to refinement of a youth-specific collaborative model for further integration of mental health and SUD treatment. The child psychiatrist, psychologist, and the licensed clinical social worker (as BHC) each have been trained in the University of Washington AIMS Center CoCM, and the practice added this patient to the practice registry to monitor rating scales and coordinate care customized for this youth. Dr Child Psychiatrist's contact with the practice by telemedicine has enhanced collaboration with the team of professionals, including the psychologist. This arrangement was further enhanced when the child psychiatrist became a consultant for a state child psychiatry access program, with which this primary care practice has registered. The program has provided further access for this particular primary care practice to child psychiatric consultation, as well as continuing education presentations for all primary care and mental health professionals.

PCBH is evidence-based,[24–26] but more flexible than CoCM in its application. Embedded psychologists provide consultation, brief treatments, and when needed, referral, for common behavioral and mental health problems seen in primary care.

These include (**Fig. 3**) problems with health behaviors that affect healthy development and, when present, chronic illness. In addition, the PCBH model provides embedded services for mental health and substance use issues, offering children and families early intervention for subclinical presentations and improved access to care for more serious concerns. The goal is to promote healthy individual and family development through prevention and early intervention. The focus is on behavior change and collaboration with primary care clinicians and others, including child psychiatrists. Patients and their families in need are identified via numerous channels, including primary care clinician referral, staff referral, patient/family self-referral, screening, and chart review. Psychologists often lead the on-site behavioral health team that includes master's-level behavioral health or substance abuse clinicians who provide brief interventions and care for common primary care behavioral health problems, with oversight and consultation by psychologists and psychiatrists.

Some psychologists implement a PCBH model through functioning exclusively as BHCs. The model emphasizes a population health approach in which the BHC provides consultation to the primary care clinician regarding their care of the patient. The BHC also provides prevention and early, brief intervention services for families, with referral to outside psychologists and child psychiatrists for those needing more intensive services.

The Focus of the Primary Care Behavioral Health Model

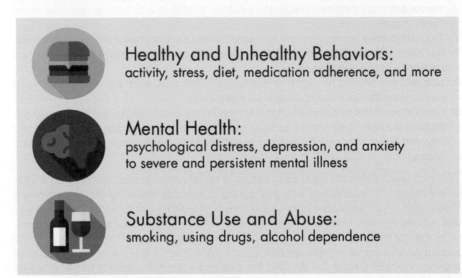

Healthy and Unhealthy Behaviors:
activity, stress, diet, medication adherence, and more

Mental Health:
psychological distress, depression, and anxiety
to severe and persistent mental illness

Substance Use and Abuse:
smoking, using drugs, alcohol dependence

Fig. 3. The focus of the PCBH model. Healthy and Unhealthy Behaviors Photo. Retrieved from APA Editorial Design Services. (Copyright © 2015 by the American Psychological Association. Reproduced with permission.)

In the PCBH example that follows, the child and family psychologist is embedded in a federally qualified health center clinic, providing a broad spectrum of services, along with a consulting child psychiatrist, a pediatric nurse practitioner (NP), and a pediatrician:

Jolita was a 16-year-old Latina, who started treatment with a psychologist for symptoms of inattention, emotional dysregulation, and increasing anxiety. The pediatrician prescribed Jolita mixed amphetamine salts for attention-deficit/hyperactivity disorder (ADHD). After Jolita's mother called because of increasing behavior problems at school, the primary care NP spoke to Jolita's pediatrician and increased the medication dose. Unfortunately, Jolita began to complain of increased anxiety and auditory hallucinations.

The psychologist called the child psychiatrist, who after reviewing the patient's history and considering possible medication effects, recommended stopping the stimulant. Jolita was medication free for 2 weeks, but her anxiety and auditory hallucinations continued. The psychologist used CBT to help Jolita manage her anxiety. She also used a family therapy approach with Jolita, her sister, and her mother to discuss witnessing of domestic violence. After this session, the child psychiatrist, assessing possible posttraumatic issues, cautiously prescribed an SSRI with follow-up with him after 2 weeks. Within a month, Jolita's anxiety was better; however, she had continued problems with the inattention that interfered with schoolwork. In psychotherapy, Jolita told the psychologist the auditory hallucinations were mainly the voice of her father, with whom she had a significantly conflictual relationship. The process reversed itself, as the psychologist used dialectical behavioral therapy and CBT strategies to increase Jolita's early awareness of symptoms of anxiety and its cues, working to include appropriate anxiety-reducing activities. During that time, her father's voice dissipated. The child psychiatrist then started Jolita on a nonstimulant for inattention; within 3 weeks, her ADHD symptoms were better controlled.

Once stable, it was agreed that the primary care NP would manage medications. In the last phase of psychotherapy, the psychologist worked directly on Jolita's relationship with her mother, coaching the mother to treat the patient like a teenager and not a friend. The mother was able to develop a confiding relationship with a friend, allowing for successful boundaries with her daughter. A year after the last therapy session, the pediatrician reported that Jolita continued to do well. He is considering a trial tapering the SSRI. (Note that if the trauma-related hallucinations had not resolved through the combination of therapy and medication intervention, the child psychiatrist was available to further assess and treat.) In this example, the relationships and communication between the primary care and embedded behavioral health professionals were essential, healing parts of the comprehensive treatment for Jolita and her family. These professionals had worked together respectfully for years, complemented each other's care, and provided excellent role models for the family. The primary care professionals wanted more help, so the team went on to grow in size and expand its services and support for this clinic.

As is illustrated in these cases, both child psychiatrists and psychologists can have roles in each model. Many larger primary care practices have instituted a blend of the CoCM and PCBH models to best serve their patients.[27] In this way, the 2 models can be complementary.

These models have increased in importance with the advent of the COVID-19 pandemic of 2020 to 2021 and its negative effect on the mental health of children, adolescents, and their families. In February 2021, *New York Times* reporter, Christina Caron, stated: *COVID creates increased demand, as well as opportunity for*

The Primary Care Behavioral Health Team in the Patient-Centered Medical Home

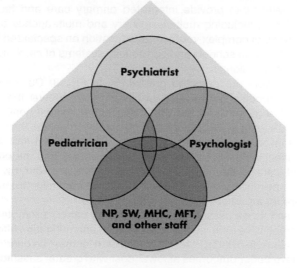

Adapted from a talk given at the Society of Developmental and Behavioral Pediatrics by Susan H McDaniel, 2020 (29)

Fig. 4. The primary care behavioral health team in the patient-centered medical home. MHC, Mental Health Counselor; MFT, Marriage & Family Therapist. (*Adapted from* a talk given at the Society of Developmental and Behavioral Pediatrics by Susan H. McDaniel, 2020.[29])

collaboration, especially after polling showed increasing presentation of patients and families with anxiety and depression. CoCM and additional forms of integrated care, including co-location models, have proven successful in meeting these challenges. Proactive screening is essential, and will require more access to care.[28] Regardless of the model used to deliver a full range of psychiatric and behavioral health services to the PCMH, any mental health professional needs to be in collaboration with, or offer access to, a full interprofessional mental health team.

Working together

As these vignettes illustrate, child psychiatrists and psychologists can and do provide mutual support and education for each other in primary care, and other contexts. Each professional is respecting, supporting, and building on the role of the other, thus moving away from competition toward building both trust and a higher level of team collaboration. Effective comprehensive care occurs through engagement by the child psychiatrist and psychologist with the primary care practice. A BHC may continue contact, behavioral support, and measurements of progress. Each model builds, albeit in different ways, the opportunity for intervention by both the psychiatrist and the psychologist. The use of blended models increases the range of care for the patient and family, and decreases tension and promotes respect among professionals.

We have much to learn from each other. In general, psychologists can continue to learn from child psychiatrists how best to screen patients for medical and psychopharmacologic issues, such as the safe use and monitoring of medications. Similarly, child psychiatrists, at times limited by traditional managed care to the role of diagnostician and medication prescriber, can expand their knowledge of behavior change and psychotherapies through closer contact with psychologists. The best leaders will, regardless of their particular profession, emerge and continue to support the other team professionals. Each profession needs coherent and well-defined professional identities and a commitment to interprofessional teamwork. Then child psychiatrists and psychologists together can provide integrated primary care and facilitate needed care in many settings, including multidisciplinary and multi-agency treatment team planning, case review of complex youth, brief education on specialized topics, collaboration with other teams in schools and community systems of care, and consultation with primary care professionals.

Overlapping skill sets are depicted graphically in **Fig. 3**. Our overlapping skills sometimes fuel competitive tensions about hierarchy and power that are harmful to both the care of the patient and the well-being of the mental health professionals and the primary care team more broadly. In collaborative practice, the skills and power of each professional are recognized, and the issues resolved and aligned for the benefit of the patient. Primary care physicians sometimes find the process of instituting integrated care a daunting task. If we understand our own professional strengths as child psychiatrists and psychologists, we can help structure and implement shared care for a particular primary care practice.

The PCMH,[30] and its successor, advanced primary care,[31] promote proactive, coordinated, comprehensive care, suited to prevention and mitigation efforts for chronic diseases through the use of interprofessional clinician teams. The quadruple aim of the PCMH is to achieve better outcomes at lower cost with greater satisfaction for the patient and the clinician. Accomplishing these aims requires that integrated care teams have good communication and clear roles, so that all members are working at the top of their licensure, training, experience, and competence. Health care has become a team sport, and as with other team sports, it can be fun, yet takes preparation, practice, and hard work. This is especially true in integrated care, in which primary care physicians collaborate with a wide variety of medical professionals; they expect the same degree of cooperation and mutual respect among the collaborating mental health professionals.

Collaborative leadership

In most medical settings, such as hospital and academic health centers, psychiatry and behavioral health programs typically have a hierarchical organizational structure, with physicians in most leadership positions. However, not infrequently, psychologists also hold clinical and administrative leadership positions. They may supervise multidisciplinary training programs, and consultation and liaison or integrated care programs in primary and specialty care. In primary care, moving from "I" (the individual practitioner) to "we" (team-based care) means that clinical leadership may be rotated, requiring information-gathering and decision-making by the professional with the most relevant skills and the strongest relationship with a particular patient and family, with the input and support of the integrated primary care team.[32] We cannot assume that we will be *the leader* of every team, although we must continue to contribute as *a leader* to each team on which we serve, seeking clinical and administrative opportunities to do so. Shared leadership with other professionals is likely to enhance and expand our own opportunities. This approach to leadership is similar to that in many current military and business contexts. At the 2014 American Association of Medical Colleges meeting, General Stanley McChrystal elaborated on this point when speaking about his experience in the US Armed Services and VA systems: *In today's world, it's the people who are humble enough and empathetic enough to listen and discern what the situation is, what's required, and then adapt themselves to that requirement, who are going to be the most effective, important leaders of the future.*[uu]

Rotating or shared collaborative leadership can be highly productive and creative, whether in clinical practice, program development, training, or research. It can also increase available services in the community. Teams of primary care clinicians, child psychiatrists, psychologists, and other professionals can serve as a leadership hub, with spokes out to peer support, community-based and home-based programs, and community agencies. In these networks, child psychiatrists and psychologists are consultants to, or partners with, NPs, social workers, counselors, pharmacists, and other specialists, as well as to preliminary degree graduates and paraprofessionals. Additional collaborative contexts include joint research, joint publication in child psychiatry and psychology journals, child psychiatry access programs, joint presentations and continuing medical education productions, and school consultation.

Improving Access and Outcomes while Invigorating Our Professions through Interprofessional Teamwork

Collaborative, integrated care by child psychiatrists and psychologists holds the potential of increasing the effectiveness and value of our respective services, while supporting better access and outcomes for our patients and their families. To do so, we need to expand on current collaborative and integrated care models; develop and evaluate new practice models that can better meet the needs of our population; transform our training models to include interprofessional education and training; and collaborate on local, state, and federal advocacy. All of these goals will be advanced by enhanced collaboration between our professional associations.

Our needed transformation in practice

To do so is both exciting, and for most, cuts against the grain of traditional training. For child psychiatrists and psychologists to work together effectively, we must

- Manage our fear of change by considering the likely possibility that the work will be rewarding, stimulating, and reduce burnout.
- See ourselves and each other as essential to the success of collaborative and integrated health care.
- Consider that sharing responsibility and leadership with traditional competitors will not "put us out of business" nor "usurp each other's areas of specialty or leadership roles." (The demand for our collaborative services far exceeds any of our capacities.)
- Seek fair and competitive reimbursement for collaborative services to incentivize and stabilize the change.
- Work toward alternate payment models that are just and favorable.

To join together in providing comprehensive primary care, we need to build relationships with each other and primary care teams based on competence, trust, and communication. Once a relationship is established, it is easier for the child psychiatrist and psychologist to discuss instituting a collaborative care practice model with the primary care practice. This may include preparing the primary care practice for embedded and consulting professionals, billing, registry, measurements, and training a BHC.

Needed transformation in training

This collaborative way of working is best learned through interprofessional education (IPE) and training, with access to models and mentors. It is worth seeking out an experienced mentor who likes interdisciplinary work, is good at tolerating uncertainty, and is able to handle the challenging presentations that occur in primary care. IPE is essential to producing psychiatrists and psychologists who know how to collaborate in transformative practice from the beginnings of their careers. This training in collaboration and teams must be built into graduate and postgraduate training so that trainees continue to move from a competitive "us and them" perspective to a collaborative "we."[34,35]

Professional associations and systems offer valuable training to child psychiatrists and psychologists. The American Psychiatric Association has trained thousands of psychiatrists in the CoCM,[36] with AACAP developing models attuned to care for youth, including child psychiatry access programs and youth-specific measurement–based care (an article in this journal addresses in detail the process of team formation.) The REACH Institute and Project Echo help to build acumen for mental health issues for primary care physicians, preparing them for integrated care. The American Psychological Association offers workshops and webinars on PCBH and specialty integrated behavioral health care. On-site and online courses exist (see Trainings at the end of this article).

Advocacy

Together, we can build financial support for our professions and our models through collective advocacy. The PCMH, and its hope for better quality care at lower cost, may retain higher proportions of risk-based payments through flexibly planned and delivered care, with behavioral health strategies fine-tuned in consultation with psychologists and child psychiatrists. Primary care consultation enhances the trust-building needed to institute an integrated care practice model. We can then jointly approach payers to cover PCBH, CoCM, expansion of coverage for COVID-19, support for post-grant sustainability of child psychiatry access programs, and enforcement of parity.

Enhancing Our Professions Through Enhanced Collaboration by Our Professional Associations

Our professional associations can work together to promote our joint missions. For example, in 2019 AACAP, AAP, Society of Child and Adolescent Psychology, Society for Developmental and Behavioral Pediatrics, and Society of Pediatric Psychology *jointly* commissioned a national study by the Milliman Group.[7] The study showed MH/SUDs in children and youth with chronic mental health conditions (CMCs) are associated with higher total health care payments for both patients and their parents, suggesting prevention or reducing the impact of MH/SUDs among youth with CMCs. Joining forces, with these data and mutual advocacy, is important to having payers and legislators listen.

The Primary Care Collaborative's Behavioral Health Integration Workgroup and the Path Forward Program promoted by the National Alliance of Healthcare Purchasers Coalition are active in encouraging programs that involve creative and effective team-building. Forward-looking payers are assessing various approaches to collaborative and integrated care delivery, funding both fee-for-service and value-based options to develop an evidence base. They monitor measurements and outcomes in both small and large practice models, and they emphasize the need for "all hands on deck" by authorizing payment for professionals with respect to their role on the integrated team.[37]

Specific collaboration between AACAP and various divisions of the American Psychological Association may include the following:

1. Liaisons between leadership and organizational components and committees.
2. Alliances within our organizations, in which a body of child psychiatrists and psychologists cooperate on areas of mutual interest.
3. Collaborative projects and products, such as joint practice parameters and policy statements. (For example, the American Psychiatric Association recently convened a group of 10 organizations, including the American Psychological Association, and produced a document of 9 key principles for interprofessional care of people with serious mental illness.[38])
4. Collaboration in development of clinical measurements and rating scales appropriate to children and adolescents.
5. Certificates of appreciation and acknowledgment.
6. Promoting and supporting training and best practice models for collaboration among child psychiatrists and psychologists.

A Vision of the Future

Those child psychiatrists and psychologists who wish to continue in private practice may want to transition at least some of their time to collaborative and integrated care. This will offer a break from traditional managed care, especially for those child psychiatrists who are inundated with brief medication visits or long inpatient hours and psychologists wishing to deliver more modes of therapy and behavioral interventions than is typical in the private office. The more that child psychiatrists are open to, work on creating, and make themselves available for, collaboration with comprehensive care teams, the more likely they will be called on as valued and essential team members.[11] The same is true for psychologists.

Team leadership and consultant roles are more likely to be flexible and engaging in transformed care than in traditional practice. Our premise is evident in our case examples presented previously; a key principle is that psychologists and child psychiatrists continue to consult and collaborate with each other in evidence-based models of comprehensive integrated primary care, as we adapt models for children and adolescents. Allocation of $80 million toward expansion of child psychiatry access programs by the recently enacted American Rescue Plan Act will facilitate development of these models.[39]

Mutual advocacy will promote the unified expertise of child psychiatrists, psychologists, and other professionals to primary care practices and payers. It will provide the innovation and joy that comes from participating in developing and implementing multidisciplinary comprehensive treatment plans that reflect ideas and strategies that can only result from collaboration beyond one's own profession. In the end, the most important question is: "Will this help the kids?" Both of us answer this with a resounding "YES!" Our hope is that this article will spur child psychiatrists and psychologists to further engagement, mutual respect, and the skill development needed to transform practice and support our patients and families, as well as our own healthy development and well-being.

DISCLOSURES

None.

REFERENCES

1. McDaniel SH, Hepworth J, Campbell TL, et al. Working together: collaboration and referral to family-oriented mental health professionals, . Family-oriented primary care. 2nd ed. New York, NY: Springer; 2005.
2. McDaniel SH, Hepworth J. Family psychology in primary care: Managing issues of power and dependency through collaboration. In: Frank R, McDaniel S, Bray J, et al, editors. American Psychological Association Publications. 2003; Washington, DC: Primary care psychology. 2004. p. 131–2.
3. Cuellar AE, Haas-Wilson D. Competition and the mental health system. Am J Psychiatry 2009;166(3):278–83.
4. Scull A. Contested jurisdictions: psychiatry, psychoanalysis, and clinical psychology in the United States, 1940-2010. Med Hist 2011;55(3):401–6.
5. Moran M. Collaborative care rises to the pandemic challenge. Psychiatr News Clin Res 2021. Available at: https://psychnews.psychiatryonline.org/doi/full/10.1176/appi.pn.2021.1.12. Accessed May 20, 2021.
6. Borer MS, Committee C-coAsHCAE. Discussion forum: summary of AACAP assembly Listserv discussion on relationships with psychologists 2016.
7. Perrin JM, Asarnow JR, Stancin T, et al. Mental health conditions and health care payments for children with chronic medical conditions. Acad Pediatr 2019;19(1):44–50.
8. Melek ST, Norris DT, Paulus J, Matthews K, Weaver A, and Davenport S. Potential economic impact of integrated medical-behavioral healthcare. Milliman Research Report, 2018.
9. American Academy of Child and Adolescent Psychiatrists. AACAP releases workforce maps illustrating severe shortage of child and adolescent psychiatrists. 2018. Available at: https://www.aacap.org/AACAP/Press/Press_Releases/2018/Severe_Shortage_of_Child_and_Adolescent_Psychiatrists_Illustrated_in_AAACP_Workforce_maps.aspx. Accessed May 20, 2021.
10. Axelson D. Beyond a bigger workforce: addressing the shortage of child and adolescent psychiatrists. 2020. Available at: https://pediatricsnationwide.org/2020/04/10/beyond-a-bigger-workforce-addressing-the-shortage-of-child-and-adolescent-psychiatrists/. Accessed May 20, 2021.
11. Thompson KS. Psychiatry and primary health care: beyond integration, toward fusion? Psychiatr Times 2016;33(7). Available at: https://www.psychiatrictimes.com/view/psychiatry-and-primary-health-care-beyond-integration-toward-fusion. Accessed: May 20, 2021.

12. Lin LL, Christidis P, Stamm K. A look at psychologists' specialty areas, Center for Workforce Studies. Monitor Psychol Datapoint 2017;48(8). Available at: https://www.apa.org/monitor/2017/09/datapoint. Accessed: May 21, 2021.

13. American Academy of Child and Adolescent Psychiatrists. Goals & recommendations (the "Roadmap") for the coming decade (2013-2023). In: Back to project future: plan for the coming decade: a Presidential Initiative of Martin J. Drell, M.D. Washington, DC: American Academy of Child and Adolescent Psychiatry; 2014. p. 15–44.

14. The Accreditation Council for Graduate Medical Education. The American Board of Psychiatry and Neurology. The Child and Adolescent Psychiatry Milestone Project, July 2015. 2015. Available at:https://www.acgme.org/portals/0/pdfs/milestones/childandadolescentpsychiatrymilestones.pdf. . 1-27. Accessed: May 20, 2021.

15. McDaniel SH, Grus CL, Cubic BA, et al. Competencies for psychology practice in primary care. Am Psychol 2014;69(4):409–29.

16. Tharp T. The collaborative habit: life lessons for working together. New York: Simon and Schuster; 2009.

17. Kazak AE. Pediatric Psychosocial Preventative Health Model (PPPHM): research, practice, and collaboration in pediatric family systems medicine. Fam Syst Health 2006;24(4):381.

18. Ader J, Stille CJ, Keller D, et al. The medical home and integrated behavioral health: advancing the policy agenda. Pediatrics 2015;135(5):909–17.

19. McDaniel SH, Campbell TL, Hepworth J, et al. Family-oriented primary care. 2nd ed. New York, NY. Springer Science & Business Media; 2005.

20. Medical Director Institute. The psychiatric shortage. causes and solutions, 27, 2017. Available at: https://www.thenationalcouncil.org/wp-content/uploads/2017/03/Psychiatric-Shortage_National-Council-.pdf?daf=375ateTbd56. Accessed February 14, 2021.

21. Ratzliff A, Unützer J, Katon W, et al. Integrated care: creating effective mental and primary health care teams. Hoboken, NJ: John Wiley & Sons; 2016.

22. Aims Center. Evidence base for COCM 2021. Available at: https://aims.uw.edu/collaborative-care/evidence-base-cocm. Accessed May 20, 2021.

23. Simon KM, Harris SK, Shrier LA, et al. Measurement-based care in the treatment of adolescents with substance use disorders. Child Adolesc Psychiatr Clin N Am 2020;29(4):675–90.

24. Asarnow JR, Rozenman M, Wiblin J, et al. Integrated medical-behavioral care compared with usual primary care for child and adolescent behavioral health: a meta-analysis. JAMA Pediatr 2015;169(10):929–37.

25. Kearney LK, Post EP, Pomerantz AS, et al. Applying the interprofessional patient aligned care team in the Department of Veterans Affairs: Transforming primary care. Am Psychol 2014;69(4):399–408.

26. Pomerantz A, Cole BH, Watts BV, et al. Improving efficiency and access to mental health care: combining integrated care and advanced access. Gen Hosp Psychiatry 2008;30(6):546–51.

27. Raney LE, Lasky GB, Scott C. Integrated care: a guide for effective implementation. Washington, DC: American Psychiatric Pub; 2017.

28. Caron C. Creating collaborative care. The New York Times 2021.

29. McDaniel SH. Communication with patients and families with developmental and behavioral problems. Paper presented at: Society for Developmental & Behavioral Pediatrics Annual Meeting; October 11, 2020; Virtual.

30. Baird M, Blount A, Brungardt S, et al. The development of joint principles: integrating behavioral health care into the patient-centered medical home. Ann Fam Med 2014;12(2):183.

31. Jabbarpour Y, Coffman M, Habib A, et al. Advanced primary care: a key contributor to successful ACOs 2018. Washington, DC. Available at: https://dhss.delaware.gov/dhss/dhcc/files/pcpevidencerpt2018.pdf.

32. Fiscella K, McDaniel SH. The complexity, diversity, and science of primary care teams. Am Psychol 2018;73(4):451–67.

33. McChrystal S. The leadership plenary. Paper presented at: Learn Serve Lead: Association of American Medical Colleges Annual Conference; 2014; Chicago, IL.

34. Rozensky RH, Grus CL, Goodie JL, et al. A curriculum for an interprofessional seminar on integrated primary care: developing competencies for interprofessional collaborative practice. J Allied Health 2018;47(3). e47, e61-e66.

35. Brashers VL, Curry CE, Harper DC, et al. Interprofessional health care education: recommendations of the National Academies of Practice expert panel on health care in the 21st century. Issues Interdiscip Care 2001;3(1):21–31.

36. American Psychiatric Association. Get trained in the collaborative care model. Integrated Care. 2021. Available at: https://www.psychiatry.org/psychiatrists/practice/professional-interests/integrated-care/get-trained. Accessed May 21, 2021.

37. Borer MS. Personal communication of psychiatry co-author with Oleg Tarkovsky, director of behavioral health services of CareFirst BlueCross BlueShield, 2021.

38. Moran M. APA, MH groups agree on principles to improve care of SMI. Psychiatr News 2021. Available at: https://doi.org/10.1176/appi.pn.2021.2.36. Accessed February 9, 2021.

39. 117th Congress (2021-2022) - 1st Session. American Rescue Plan Act of 2021; Congressional Record Vol. 167, No. 48. 2021. Daily: Available at:https://www.congress.gov/congressional-record/2021/3/15/senate-section/article/s1510-1?q=%7B%22search%22%3A%5B%22American+Rescue+Plan%22%5D%7D&s=1&r=1. . Accessed May 21, 2021.

Effective Partnership Care Models with Advanced Practice Psychiatric Nurses

Suzie C. Nelson, MD[a],*, Jessica K. Jeffrey, MD, MBA, MPH[b],
Andrew Lustbader, MD[c], Jessica Rak, MSN[d], Mona Gandhi, MSN[d],
Rajeev Krishna, MD, PhD[e], Marcus Merriman, MS[e],
Vonda Keels-Lowe, MSN[e], Amy Hoisington-Stabile, MD[e]

KEYWORDS

- Advanced practice psychiatric nursing • Advanced practice registered nurse
- Child and adolescent psychiatrist • Collaboration
- Psychiatric mental health nurse practitioner • Scope of practice

KEY POINTS

- Workforce shortages of all mental health professionals, including child and adolescent psychiatrists, contribute to a public health crisis.
- Advanced practice psychiatric nurses, and more specifically and recently, psychiatric mental health nurse practitioners (PMHNPs), are available as a professional group that can address the workforce shortages.
- Lack of understanding of the scope of practice for PMHNPs and confusion about regulation can contribute to conflict and interfere with collaborative practice.
- Several models of effective collaborations between child and adolescent psychiatrists and PMHNPs are presented for consideration.

[a] Wright State University Boonshoft School of Medicine Department of Psychiatry, 2555 University Boulevard, Dayton, OH 45324, USA; [b] Department of Psychiatry & Biobehavioral Sciences, Division of Population Behavioral Health, Semel Institute for Neuroscience and Human Behavior, UCLA, 760 Westwood Plaza, A7-372A, Los Angeles, CA 90095, USA; [c] Child Guidance Center of Mid-Fairfield County, 215 Main Street, Westport, CT 06880, USA; [d] Child Guidance Center of Mid-Fairfield County, Clinical instructor Yale School of Nursing, 100 East Avenue, Norwalk, CT 06851, USA; [e] Department of Psychiatry, Nationwide Children's Hospital, 444 Butterfly Garden's Drive, Columbus, OH 43215, USA
* Corresponding author.
E-mail address: Suzie.nelson@wright.edu

Child Adolesc Psychiatric Clin N Am 30 (2021) 827–838
https://doi.org/10.1016/j.chc.2021.07.005
1056-4993/21/© 2021 Elsevier Inc. All rights reserved.

Abbreviations	
APPNs	Advanced practice psychiatric nurses
APN	Advanced practice nurse
APRNs	Advanced practice registered nurses
CAPs	Child and adolescent psychiatrists
EDT	Extended day treatment
IOPs	Intensive outpatient programs
NP	Nurse practitioner
PMHNPs	Psychiatric mental health nurse practitioners

INTRODUCTION

Within the United States, approximately 15 million children and adolescents suffer from behavioral health disorders.[1] Behavioral health disorders in childhood compromise cognitive, social, and emotional development and contribute to lifelong disability.[2] Unfortunately, only 20% of children and adolescents with behavioral health symptoms receive treatment.[3] This creates a huge public health crisis, as the vast majority of children and adolescents with behavioral health disorders do not receive the treatment they need.[4]

While this public health burden is multifactorial in etiology, substantial contributors are the longstanding shortage and inequitable distribution of child and adolescent psychiatrists (CAPs), who generally live and practice in larger and more affluent cities.[5] There are approximately 9950 practicing child and adolescent psychiatrists in the United States,[6] which equates to approximately one child and adolescent psychiatrist per 1500 children in need of services. Compounding the issue, children in rural areas have reduced access compared with those in urban areas. The ratio of child and adolescent psychiatrists per 100,000 people ranges from 1.3 in Idaho to 11.4 in the District of Columbia.[6] Further, CAPs are often involved in the care of transitional age youth, and while the increasing number of insured young adults is an overall positive development in health care reform, all mental health providers struggle to meet the increased legitimate demand for services that the growing insured population represents.[7]

In order to address the dearth of CAPs, the field has supported training pediatric primary care practitioners to screen, diagnose, and treat common behavioral health conditions. Additionally, behavioral health integration within primary care has been explored and promoted.[8] Previous research has proposed the ongoing shortage in the psychiatric workforce may be at least partly remedied by advanced practice psychiatric nurses.[9] Historically, CAPs have adopted critical roles of guiding nurse practitioners' education in pediatric behavioral health and provided support to these valuable professionals. However, variable requirements across states, reimbursement issues, and liability concerns are among the barriers suggesting that compulsory regulation of these historical care models is not sustainable.

Enhanced partnerships with other care providers, such as nurse practitioners, will be an essential step in addressing these known workforce challenges that have failed to fill the access to care gaps for children and adolescents with behavioral health conditions. While cooperation among physicians and advanced practice registered nurses (APRNs) are seen across specialties and in primary care, we will focus specifically on the importance of partnerships between CAPs and psychiatric mental health nurse practitioners (PMHNPs), or more broadly, advanced practice psychiatric nurses (APPNs). We examine the current state of PMHNP practice and models of effective care management among CAPs and PMHNPs that show promise to meet these needs for vulnerable youth.

ROLES AND DEFINITIONS

Little has been published specifically about PMHNPs who primarily treat children and adolescents. A systematic review on the role performance of APRNs revealed that they perform multifaceted roles and provide behavioral health services in a variety of contexts, including outpatient, inpatient, and emergency department settings.[9] Most studies have examined the impact of psychosocial interventions. The paper describes favorable outcomes for patients with depression and psychological stress in outpatient settings when advanced practice nurses were involved in the provision of psychosocial interventions. The settings reviewed included adult primary and subspecialty-care settings, older adults' domiciles, and a private practice setting. The review included one study with adolescents. Specifically, Hardin and colleagues revealed the positive impact of a psychological intervention conducted by APRN on 1030 adolescents exposed to a hurricane.[10]

Other roles described in the paper included nurse-directed services in health care contexts. Results generally demonstrated improvement in care for psychiatric inpatients and in the emergency department. One study reported insignificant results when nurses conducted transitional care for patients with schizophrenia or schizoaffective disorder who were being discharged from a psychiatric hospital. Lastly, psychiatric advance practice nurses were determined to contribute to positive patient outcomes when working with non-mental-health professionals.[9] Fairman and colleagues conclude their review provides preliminary evidence that advanced practice nurses attain positive results when working with patients with depression and psychological stress.[9]

In an examination of the global emergence of the APRN career field, this group of professionals developed from goals to improve access to medical care by reducing wait times, reducing costs, serving underprivileged patients, and maintaining health in certain populations. The United States has the longest history of the APRN career field.[11] However, roles, responsibilities, and limitations are not clearly understood or defined. This may be due to a lack of understanding about the education and training of APRNs and confusion about regulations that guide practice.

TRAINING AND CURRENT REGULATIONS
Training

Historically, the psychiatric mental health advanced practice nurse (PMH APN) has been a part of the health professional community for more than 60 years. First licensed and certified as clinical nurse specialists (PMH CNSs), this has always been a registered nurse with an additional graduate degree. Nurse practitioner (NP) pathways emerged later and gained greater recognition among colleagues and patients, so in 2001 PMH CNS graduate pathways became more aligned with PMHNP ones. Both are considered PMH APNs, although the PMH CNS educational pathways are no longer available today.[12] While both PMH APN types can be direct care professionals, 9 states still restrict prescribing by PMH CNSs.[13] PMHNPs have prescribing privileges in all 50 states and the District of Columbia.[14]

Educational and certification pathways are shown in **Fig. 1**.[14] Of note, while a doctorate-level graduate degree is not required for certification, encouragement toward earning a doctorate has grown over the last 10 years. All graduate-level work for PMHNPs focuses on areas such as pathophysiology, pharmacology, psychiatry,

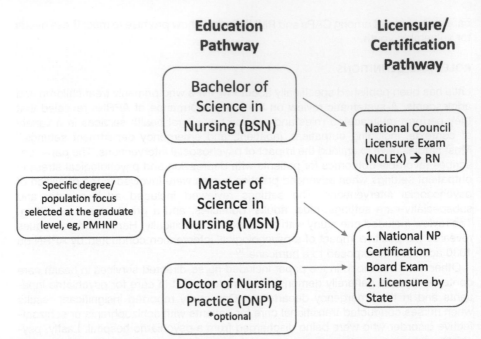

Education Pathway

Licensure/Certification Pathway

Bachelor of Science in Nursing (BSN)

National Council Licensure Exam (NCLEX) → RN

Specific degree/population focus selected at the graduate level, eg, PMHNP

Master of Science in Nursing (MSN)

1. National NP Certification Board Exam
2. Licensure by State

Doctor of Nursing Practice (DNP)
*optional

Fig. 1. Educational and certification pathways for advanced practice registered nurses (APRNs). Updated November 10, 2020. (Source American Association of Nurse Practitioners.)

neuroscience, and psychotherapy. Upon graduation and board certification, PMHNPs have been educated to conduct assessments, formulate treatment plans, prescribe medications, and participate in various systems of care.[12]

Regulations on Practice

As summarized in **Table 1**,[14] there are significant differences in defined scopes of practice among APRNs, including PMHNPs, based on state regulations, ultimately placing the control with state legislatures over state licensing boards. These differences stand in stark contrast to the recommendation that "nurses should practice to the full extent of their education and training" (IOM 2011).[15] This broad and sweeping recommendation and its corollaries have national practice implications, yet mental health practice and access to critical mental health care depend on state regulations that vary widely. While there are limited studies examining the effect of varying regulations on PMHNPs in particular, Phoenix and Chapman embarked on a series of qualitative studies examining experiences of PMHNPs in various states with differing regulations on practice and discovered interesting and consistent themes following interviews with PMHNPs and psychiatrists. These themes may shed light on the importance of the IOM recommendation from a decade ago.

APRN contribution to address workforce shortages has already been demonstrated to increase access to quality care, particularly in areas where it has been historically difficult to recruit physicians, including rural areas and in areas of low socioeconomic status.[16] One obvious way in which differing regulations across state lines create confusion and limitations on practice is when large metropolitan areas span geographically over multiple states with regulations that differ among the states but with the same mental health agency serving the entire area. Differing state regulations can also negatively impact telehealth practice if the mental health professional must

Table 1
Practice Environment Details describing practice permissions or limitations of nurse practitioners for each of the United States and the District of Columbia. Updated January 1, 2021

Practice Environment	Full Practice	Reduced Practice	Restricted Practice
Regulations/ Characteristics of Practice	Evaluation, Diagnosis, Assessment, Prescribing Authority	Reduced ability in at least one area or setting of practice. Career-long collaborative agreement required.	Restricted ability in at least one area or setting of practice. Career-long supervision required.
States	Alaska Arizona Colorado Connecticut District of Columbia Hawaii Idaho Iowa Maine Maryland Massachusetts Minnesota Montana Nebraska Nevada New Hampshire New Mexico North Dakota Oregon Rhode Island South Dakota Vermont Washington Wyoming	Alabama Arkansas Delaware Illinois Indiana Kansas Kentucky Louisiana Mississippi New Jersey New York Ohio Pennsylvania Utah West Virginia Wisconsin	California Florida Georgia Michigan Missouri North Carolina Oklahoma South Carolina Tennessee Texas Virginia

Source: American Association of Nurse Practitioners.

meet differing supervisory requirements for one group of patients versus another. States with stricter limitations of APRN practice have difficulty recruiting PMHNPs, and when this circumstance intersects with both limitations of CAP supply and larger areas of low socioeconomic status, the differential distribution of access to mental health care becomes painfully obvious. Other themes that emerged included greater overall confusion about regulatory requirements in states with stricter limitations on APRN practice and some cases wherein the PMHNP had difficulty finding quality supervision by a psychiatrist or physician attrition resulted in sudden disruptions in the ability of the PMHNP to continue practice with an established panel of patients. The greater the regulation, the greater the administrative burden for both the PMHNP and the psychiatrist, with duties such as meetings and documentation cosignature taking away from both professionals' abilities to see more patients.[17–20] Mandated supervision or mandated collaborative agreements varied both in quality for the APRN and could vary widely in monetary cost to the APRN.[21]

Successful partnerships between PMHNPs and psychiatrists were ones in which the professionals freely agreed to work together rather than being under a compulsory and regulated collaboration with greater administrative burden. These collegial professional relationships invited colleagues with shared clinical interests to work together, and parties gleaned mutual benefit.[17]

PARTNERSHIP CARE MODELS
Inpatient Psychiatric Unit

Inpatient psychiatric services offer a unique opportunity for the implementation of inter-professional care models between PMHNPs and CAPs. While ambulatory psychiatric care frequently involves individual patient assessment and offline care coordination, the inpatient setting naturally lends itself to opportunities for direct and dynamic engagement on the same patient population. A major challenge in such settings is ensuring that each practitioner is able to maximize the scope and efficiency of practice by using collaborative efforts to improve rather than duplicate care.

A shared workload model is one way to maximize this multidisciplinary model. A group of patients is supported by a PMHNP who serves as the primary provider level liaison between members of the multidisciplinary team. The PMHNP operates in the full scope of practice, taking on responsibility for treatment planning and day-to-day care management, including independent assessment and family collaboration and coordination. A CAP also sees all patients on the team and provides active shared responsibilities with the PMHNP. The CAP is responsible for validating the clinical impression and treatment direction of the team and is ultimately responsible for ensuring that the treatment plan is correct and that the treatment ultimately delivered is appropriate.

Day-to-day management is completed by the PMHNP, enabling the CAP time to focus on particularly complex cases or other areas of practice. For example, while a PMHNP would cover a single team, a full-time clinical workload for the CAP would be to cover 2 teams (each with a PMHNP), or one team and other comparable clinical or administrative responsibilities. The model also allows the CAP to provide added support when needed without disrupting the overall flow, such as when building experience and capacity in a newly graduated PMHNP.

The key to making this collegial care model successful has been a culture of mutual communication and respect. Each profession must respect the skill and training of the other, nurturing growth with a goal of building shared capacity over time. With a skilled PMHNP and CAP, the end result is less a formal "consulting" or "supervisory" relationship but rather a sharing of the total work of patient care. One day, the CAP may spend extra time evaluating a complicated catatonic patient with medical comorbidities, briefly checking in on a more standard depressed patient to ensure that they have a good understanding of the case, while the PMHNP follows up on specific needs for the catatonic patient and does an extensive workup on the depressed patient and initiates CBT. The next day, the PMHNP may spend time working with the families of both patients while the CAP attends to a separate administrative responsibility, comfortable in the knowledge that the care needs of the patients and families on the team are being well met.

Extended Day Treatment

Within this model, the PMHNP works as part of a multidisciplinary team to provide psychiatric support for children and their families. In one model of this type of clinical setting, a PMHNP is able to work with the medical director, and the caseload is divided between the 2 providers based on availability. As this is typically a part-time position for both the medical director and the PMHNP, the addition of a PMHNP affords both partners more time to be present at the clinic. In some cases, promotion to associate medical director is afforded a PMHNP, speaking to the level of respect and authority that is held within particular teams of psychiatrists and PMHNPs.

Teamwork in the EDT at this elevated level of clinical care is emphasized in weekly treatment team meetings wherein formulations and dialogue occur about guiding the treatment for each child. Psychoeducation among the team members and with the family/child ensures there is a clear understanding of the diagnosis and how treatment is addressing all areas of the patient's life, including how the family is supported, how the patient is supported individually, and how the patient interacts with and is supported by the school system and community. The PMHNP is typically on call 24/7 for any urgent matters due to the acuity of the caseload, and if there are any hospitalizations, the PMHNP will ensure that dialogue occurs between the medical director and clinical director. The PMHNP invests an hour weekly to observe patients in the group setting and will at times attend family meetings. The PMHNP role affords the combination of autonomy and leadership similar to that given to the psychiatrist in guiding treatment and making recommendations, as well as weekly and ongoing engagement and support from the medical director and the interdisciplinary team. Having the direct care staff and/or clinician participating in most medication management sessions supports this further. Finally, as the child is discharged to a more typical outpatient setting, the PMHNP may continue providing psychiatric bridge care to ensure continuity and act as a transitional object for the patient and family as they are stepping down from EDT to weekly therapy.

In other more intensive services, such as intensive in-home child and adolescent psychiatric services or other intensive outpatient programs (IOPs), PMHNPs can provide the psychiatric evaluations and medication back up for all of these programs and are used within the medical model, often hired by the agency to work with the medical director of the program but to manage all cases independent of the psychiatrist. As explained above, the role affords more child and adolescent psychiatric coverage for children in higher need throughout the various levels of care.

Outpatient Practice

In some private practice settings, PMHNPs have the ability to work within the context of a group but remain independent practitioners with a contract with the psychiatrist who owns the practice. In this case there is an employment agreement, along with a payment plan that affords the psychiatrist a base rate for each client seen. Therefore, as the PMHNP increases caseload and sees more patients, more money is provided to the practice. While at times there is a balance to determine if this is financially advantageous compared to the PMHNP opening their own independent practice, investment in the practice offsets overhead costs, such as administrative and billing staff.

Within a private practice that includes multiple mental health professional disciplines, including psychologists and social workers, teamwork is more natural. Based on the framework of the practice, there are opportunities for collegial engagement within that lens, including case discussions using a psychodynamic framework on a weekly basis. Additionally, the PMHNP can pursue other trainings in areas of interest to bring into the practice to create the independent practice that is most suitable for that APRN. Depending on the availability, in a private practice, the PMHNP can have a caseload of active therapy clients, while providing medication management in combination treatment.

In another outpatient setting, typically the CAP and the APRN maintain caseloads independent of one another, but for more challenging or complex cases, the treatment team works collaboratively to coordinate the management of patient care. The CAP and APRN discuss their cases, the approach to best manage medications if warranted, and review the complete therapeutic needs of the child and family. All mental health professionals on the treatment team work together to develop a formal case conceptualization and a clear treatment plan, and recommendations stem from this collaborative effort. The psychiatrist respects the autonomy of the APN as a provider of care. Management of complex cases using this team-based approach builds trust and mutual respect as well as ongoing professional development in practice. Successful collaboration between professionals on the treatment team requires a clear definition and understanding of roles. Communication must be clear in order to be successful. Engagement can be further increased by adopting an open-minded approach, which is positive, curious, and boosts creativity with fresh and diverse ideas. This promotes a better understanding of each professional's respective contributions and facilitates a "can do" stance. Adopting a team vision in this particular outpatient practice simplifies goal setting by recognizing individual strengths and establishing achievable milestones.

Behavioral Health Integration into Pediatric Practice

PMHNPs are also used within the medical home model of pediatric practices. The practice had already embraced the necessity of paralleling health care while addressing psychosocial issues. The pediatric practice had already utilized the services of a social worker who does family and individual counseling, as well as having a neuropsychologist available for psychological testing on a contract basis. The practice also had a pediatric APRN who handled the ongoing maintenance of routine cases of primary ADHD within the practice. What the pediatric practice lacked was the ability to integrate comprehensive mental health evaluation, triage, and treatment of more routine mental health problems common to a general pediatric practice. Efforts to triage patients to community mental health resources were ineffective due to lack of access to care or nonadherence with follow-up and the consequent worsening of symptoms for many children.

In this model, if a pediatrician or pediatric NP notices that a patient is struggling with an issue requiring more psychiatric support, they will refer to the PMHNP embedded within the pediatric practice. In this role, a PMHNP can provide further assessment and engage in briefer treatment for less acute patients, whose mental health care ultimately remains within the pediatric practice, or they can help refer to outpatient CAPs in the community. Treatment in this case can be multimodal due to the expertise of the PMHNP. As an example, the pediatric professional may observe that a child arrives consistently anxious, the parents report they cannot sleep alone, and there have been multiple visits to the school nurse without general medical illness present. In this case, the PMHNP may be able to assess and treat symptoms of anxiety by providing shorter-term cognitive behavioral therapy without having to refer the child to an outside provider. Communication with the pediatric professional in a consultative model continues to resolution of the mental health symptoms or to a referral if symptoms worsen to the point of requiring ongoing specialty care. Known benefits of this model include reduced stigma as the child and family receive mental health intervention in the pediatric office, review of a shared electronic medical record to ensure no underlying general medical conditions are present and expedited access to mental health services. If this occurs in a setting where collaborative agreement or supervision is required by regulation, this can occur with a CAP.

Military Outpatient Mental Health Clinic

PMHNPs in military practices are fully independent, in some cases alongside psychiatrists but in other cases without a psychiatrist physically colocated within the practice. Much of the time, if a PMHNP is newly out of training, there will be a period of additional peer review by another mental health prescribing professional, whether that is a more senior PMHNP or a psychiatrist. In larger clinics where psychiatrists and PMHNPs work together, mutual respect, teamwork, and cooperation predominate the practice environment. While prescribing professionals have separate caseloads and practice independently alongside each other, the collegial atmosphere often leads to voluntary consultative discussions when there are particularly challenging cases. These discussions can be bi-directional, with the psychiatrist and PMHNP in some settings being of equal likelihood to ask the other about management in these challenging situations; in these cases, the expertise being sought is about the colleague's prior experiences rather than any implication that one professional is higher than the other.

DISCUSSION

A decade after the IOM recommendation that nurses should practice to the full extent of their education and training, with implications of a national standard that APRNs, including PMHNPs, possess the education, training, and in many cases, the experience to choose to work in partnerships with a variety of mental health professionals, we present models of relationships in a variety of treatment settings. Systems that encourage recruitment into both CAP practice and PMHNP practice will increase the workforce necessary to provide better access to care. Systems that subsequently allow these prescribing mental health professionals to distribute more evenly toward areas with very limited access will be critical to meet needs in increasingly more vulnerable youth. Multidisciplinary contact and care delivery that is practiced in training settings encourages collaborative efforts among mental health professionals.

The trend has been moving toward, rather than away from, independent practice for nurse practitioners. In 2008, 15 states allowed full independent practice without regulated collaborative agreements or supervision; as of the beginning of this calendar year, this is the practice environment in 23 states and the District of Columbia.[14] One older study examining practice patterns indicates that psychiatrists and APPNs demonstrate similarities in prescribing patterns rather than significant differences.[22] Several studies in the United States and one in the United Kingdom demonstrate similar levels of competence when comparing APRNs to psychiatrists.[22-25]

Concerns among APRNs are that restrictive patterns of supervision prevent them from practicing within their full scope. The controversy between prescribing mental health professionals is the definition of appropriate scopes of practice. The question lies in whether an APRN practicing independently is within or outside of their scope of practice, with an implication that there may be patient safety compromises if someone is practicing outside of their scope. Ultimately scope of practice has historically been defined by the individual professional in question. Any mental health professional without appropriate training in a given assessment or treatment modality who practices that modality under the guise of appropriate training and expertise is not practicing within their scope, raising concerns about safe and ethical practice. A standard of practice is to know one's practice limitations and seek consultation when needed, including when a given clinical severity level or indicated modality of treatment requires such consultation. Additional training to augment current practice with a new modality is commonly sought to add skills to the current scope of practice. This would be true for any licensed and credentialed mental health professional regardless of specific credentials.

We have presented several practice models above, occurring in differing regions and at differing levels of patient care. Among the differences in the environments in which these practice models occur is that the state regulatory requirements are not the same, with some situations in which PMHNPs practice with full independence and no supervisory or formal collaborative agreement requirements. What is similar among the models described and practiced by groups of CAPs and PMHNPs is that no matter the specific state regulatory environment, cooperation and teamwork are chief among the values held within these practices. Cooperation is the art of joining people together to accomplish a given task. Organized, engaged teams with vision, adept at communication, become empowered to overcome any challenge through mutual respect and shared effort. The overarching goal remains the same—a positive outcome not only for the child and the family but also for the CAP and PMHNP caring for the family in an ongoing partnership. Even when mental health professionals do not practice in teams on a daily basis or when there is relative geographic isolation, professional isolation is not ideal, and voluntary partnerships with colleagues provide vital opportunities to maintain currency, engage in self-care, and connect to meet challenges.

SUMMARY

Collegial partnerships among mental health professionals are a more effective way for CAPs and PMHNPs to address the public health crisis among vulnerable youth who need but cannot access treatment. Lack of understanding of backgrounds and roles between groups of professional colleagues and some of the poorly defined regulations that create an administrative burden for both professions contribute to conflict that does not foster true cooperation. There is a growing trend toward greater independence of practice for PMHNPs, and this is likely to progress because of the barriers to care that are currently created by more strict regulatory requirements. Embracing effective coordinated care models enables mental health professionals to work together to reach the same goal of better mental health care for youth and families.

CLINICS CARE POINTS

- It is beneficial for all mental health and other medical professionals to be familiar with the historical development, education and training, and regulatory policies that guide colleagues of other disciplines.
- Advocacy efforts regarding local, state, and national governance of medical care should examine the evidence base; consider that regulatory requirements may impede the progress toward greater access to mental health care, and that this could occur in disparate ways such that more vulnerable populations could continue to face barriers to care.
- CAPs and PMHNPs benefit from mutually agreeable models of interprofessional practice.

ACKNOWLEDGMENT

The authors would like to thank the American Association of Nurse Practitioners for contributing valuable reviewer feedback for this article. We also thank Amy K. Roberts, DNP, APRN, PMHNP-BC, for serving as a guest reviewer for this article.

DISCLOSURE

The corresponding author is an employee of the Department of Defense; views expressed in this article are those of the authors alone and do not represent the views of the United States Air Force, Department of Defense, or United States government. The authors have no further disclosures.

REFERENCES

1. Perou R, Bitsko RH, Blumberg SJ, et al. Mental health surveillance among children – United States, 2005—2011. MMWR 2013;62(Suppl):1–35.
2. National Research Council and Institute of Medicine. Preventing mental, emotional, and behavioral disorders among young people: progress and possibilities. Committee on prevention of mental disorders and substance Abuse among children, youth, and young adults: research and promising interventions. Washington, DC: The National Academies Press; 2009.
3. US Department of Health Human Services. Mental health: a report of the surgeon general. Rockville, MD: US Department of Health and Human Services, Substance Abuse and Mental Health Services Administration, Center for Mental Health Services, National Institutes of Health, National Institute of Mental Health; 1999.
4. Whitney D, Peterson M. US national and state-level prevalence of mental health disorders and disparities of mental health care Use in children. JAMA Pediatr 2019 Apr;173(4):389–91.
5. McBain RK, Kofner A, Stein BD, et al. Growth and distribution of child psychiatrists in the United States: 2007–2016. Pediatrics 2019;4:e20191576.
6. University of Michigan Behavioral Health Workforce Research Center. Estimating the distribution of the U.S. Psychiatric subspecialist workforce. Ann Arbor, MI: UMSPH; 2018.
7. Saloner B, Lê Cook B. An ACA provision increased treatment for young adults with possible mental illnesses relative to comparison group. Health Aff (Millwood) 2014;33(8):1425–34.
8. Walter HJ, Vernacuhlo I, Trudell EK, et al. Five-year outcomes of behavioral health integration in pediatric primary care. Pediatrics 2019;144(1):e20183243.
9. Fairman JA, Rowe JW, Hassmiller S, et al. Broadening the scope of nursing practice. N Engl J Med 2011;364(3):193–6.
10. Hardin SB, Weinrich S, Weinrich M, et al. Effects of a long-term psychosocial nursing intervention on adolescents exposed to catastrophic stress. Issues Ment Health Nurs 2002;23(6):537–51.
11. Sheer B, Wong FKY. The development of advanced nursing practice globally. J Nurs Scholarship 2008;40:204–11.
12. Delaney KR. Psychiatric mental health nursing advance practice workforce: capacity to address shortages of mental health professionals. Psychiatr Serv 2017;68(9):952–4.
13. National Association of Clinical Nurse Specialists. Scope of practice CNS independent prescriptive Authority. Available at: nacns.org/advocacy-policy/policies-affecting-cnss/scope-of-practice/. Accessed July 9, 2021.
14. American Association of Nurse Practitioners. The path to becoming a nurse practitioner (NP). Available at: aanp.org/news-feed/explote-the-variety-of-career-paths-for-nurse-practitioners. Accessed July 9, 2021.
15. Institute of Medicine. The future of nursing: leading Change, advancing health. Washington DC: The National Academies Press; 2011.
16. Buerhaus PI, DesRoches CM, Dittus R, et al. Practice characteristics of primary care nurse practitioners and physicians. Nurs Outlook 2015;63(2):144–53.

17. Phoenix BJ, Chapman SA. Effect of state regulatory environments on advanced psychiatric nursing practice. Arch Psychiatr Nurs 2020;34:370–6.
18. Chapman SA, Phoenix BJ, Hahn TE, et al. Utilization and economic contribution of psychiatric mental health nurse practitioners in public behavioral health services. Am J Prev Med 2018;54(6S3):S243–9.
19. Chapman SA, Toretsky C, Phoenix BJ. Enhancing psychiatric mental health nurse practitioner practice: impact of state scope of practice regulations. J Nurs Regul 2019;10(1):35–43.
20. Phoenix BJ, Hurd M, Chapman SA. Experience of psychiatric mental health nurse practitioners in public mental health. Nurs Adm Q 2016;40(3):212–24.
21. Martin B, Phoenix B, ChapmanS. How collaborative practice agreements impede the provision of vital behavioral health services. Nurs Outlook 2020; 19(S0029–6554):30762–6.
22. Feldman S, Bachman J, Cuffel B, et al. Advanced practice psychiatric nurses as a treatment resource: Survey and analysis. Adm Policy Ment Health Ment Health Serv Res 2003;30:479–92.
23. Fisher SE, Vaughan-Cole B. Similarities and differences in clients treated and in medications prescribed by APRNs and psychiatrists in a CMHC. Arch Psychiatr Nurs 2003;17(3):101–7.
24. Jacobs JT. Treatment of depressive disorders in split versus integrated therapy and comparisons of prescriptive practices of psychiatrists and advanced practice registered nurses. Arch Psychiatr Nurs 2005;19(6):256–63.
25. Norman IJ, While A, Whittlesea C, et al. Evaluation of mental health nurses' supplementary prescribing: final report to the department of health (England) Kings College. London: Division of Health & Social Care Research; 2007.

UNITED STATES POSTAL SERVICE® Statement of Ownership, Management, and Circulation (All Periodicals Publications Except Requester Publications)

1. Publication Title	2. Publication Number	3. Filing Date
CHILD AND ADOLESCENT PSYCHIATRIC CLINICS OF NORTH AMERICA	011 – 368	9/18/2021

4. Issue Frequency	5. Number of Issues Published Annually	6. Annual Subscriber Price
JAN, APR, JUL, OCT	4	$348.00

7. Complete Mailing Address of Known Office of Publication (Not printer) (Street, city, county, state, and ZIP+4®)

ELSEVIER INC.
230 Park Avenue, Suite 800
New York, NY 10169

Contact Person
Malathi Samayan
Telephone (Include area code)
91-44-42994507

8. Complete Mailing Address of Headquarters or General Business Office of Publisher (Not printer)

ELSEVIER INC.
230 Park Avenue, Suite 800
New York, NY 10169

9. Full Names and Complete Mailing Addresses of Publisher, Editor, and Managing Editor (Do not leave blank)

Publisher (Name and complete mailing address)

DOLORES MELONI, ELSEVIER INC.
1600 JOHN F KENNEDY BLVD. SUITE 1800
PHILADELPHIA, PA 19103-2899

Editor (Name and complete mailing address)

LAUREN BOYLE, ELSEVIER INC.
1600 JOHN F KENNEDY BLVD. SUITE 1800
PHILADELPHIA, PA 19103-2899

Managing Editor (Name and complete mailing address)

PATRICK MANLEY, ELSEVIER INC.
1600 JOHN F KENNEDY BLVD. SUITE 1800
PHILADELPHIA, PA 19103-2899

10. Owner (Do not leave blank. If the publication is owned by a corporation, give the name and address of the corporation immediately followed by the names and addresses of all stockholders owning or holding 1 percent or more of the total amount of stock. If not owned by a corporation, give the names and addresses of the individual owners. If owned by a partnership or other unincorporated firm, give its name and address as well as those of each individual owner. If the publication is published by a nonprofit organization, give its name and address.)

Full Name	Complete Mailing Address
WHOLLY OWNED SUBSIDIARY OF REED/ELSEVIER, US HOLDINGS	1600 JOHN F KENNEDY BLVD. SUITE 1800 PHILADELPHIA, PA 19103-2899

11. Known Bondholders, Mortgagees, and Other Security Holders Owning or Holding 1 Percent or More of Total Amount of Bonds, Mortgages, or Other Securities. If none, check box ▶ ☐ None

Full Name	Complete Mailing Address
N/A	

12. Tax Status (For completion by nonprofit organizations authorized to mail at nonprofit rates) (Check one)
The purpose, function, and nonprofit status of this organization and the exempt status for federal income tax purposes:
☒ Has Not Changed During Preceding 12 Months
☐ Has Changed During Preceding 12 Months (Publisher must submit explanation of change with this statement)

PS Form 3526, July 2014 [Page 1 of 4 (see instructions page 4)] PSN: 7530-01-000-9931 PRIVACY NOTICE: See our privacy policy on www.usps.com.

13. Publication Title	14. Issue Date for Circulation Data Below
CHILD AND ADOLESCENT PSYCHIATRIC CLINICS OF NORTH AMERICA	JULY 2021

15. Extent and Nature of Circulation		Average No. Copies Each Issue During Preceding 12 Months	No. Copies of Single Issue Published Nearest to Filing Date
a. Total Number of Copies (Net press run)		148	144
b. Paid Circulation (By Mail and Outside the Mail)	(1) Mailed Outside-County Paid Subscriptions Stated on PS Form 3541 (Include paid distribution above nominal rate, advertiser's proof copies, and exchange copies)	89	84
	(2) Mailed In-County Paid Subscriptions Stated on PS Form 3541 (Include paid distribution above nominal rate, advertiser's proof copies, and exchange copies)	0	0
	(3) Paid Distribution Outside the Mails Including Sales Through Dealers and Carriers, Street Vendors, Counter Sales, and Other Paid Distribution Outside USPS®	25	26
	(4) Paid Distribution by Other Classes of Mail Through the USPS (e.g., First-Class Mail®)	0	0
c. Total Paid Distribution (Sum of 15b (1), (2), (3), and (4))	▶	114	110
d. Free or Nominal Rate Distribution (By Mail and Outside the Mail)	(1) Free or Nominal Rate Outside-County Copies included on PS Form 3541	17	16
	(2) Free or Nominal Rate In-County Copies Included on PS Form 3541	0	0
	(3) Free or Nominal Rate Copies Mailed at Other Classes Through the USPS (e.g., First-Class Mail)	0	0
	(4) Free or Nominal Rate Distribution Outside the Mail (Carriers or other means)	0	0
e. Total Free or Nominal Rate Distribution (Sum of 15d (1), (2), (3) and (4))	▶	17	16
f. Total Distribution (Sum of 15c and 15e)	▶	131	126
g. Copies not Distributed (See Instructions to Publishers #4 (page 43))	▶	17	18
h. Total (Sum of 15f and g)	▶	148	144
i. Percent Paid (15c divided by 15f times 100)	▶	87.02%	87.3%

* If you are claiming electronic copies, go to line 16 on page 3. If you are not claiming electronic copies, skip to line 17 on page 3.

16. Electronic Copy Circulation		Average No. Copies Each Issue During Preceding 12 Months	No. Copies of Single Issue Published Nearest to Filing Date
a. Paid Electronic Copies	▶		
b. Total Paid Print Copies (Line 15c) + Paid Electronic Copies (Line 16a)	▶		
c. Total Print Distribution (Line 15f) + Paid Electronic Copies (Line 16a)	▶		
d. Percent Paid (Both Print & Electronic Copies) (16b divided by 16c × 100)	▶		

☒ I certify that 50% of all my distributed copies (electronic and print) are paid above a nominal price.

17. Publication of Statement of Ownership

☒ If the publication is a general publication, publication of this statement is required. Will be printed in the OCTOBER 2021 issue of this publication. ☐ Publication not required.

18. Signature and Title of Editor, Publisher, Business Manager, or Owner

Malathi Samayan Malathi Samayan, - Distribution Controller

Date 9/18/2021

I certify that all information furnished on this form is true and complete. I understand that anyone who furnishes false or misleading information on this form or who omits material or information requested on the form may be subject to criminal sanctions (including fines and imprisonment) and/or civil sanctions (including civil penalties).

PS Form 3526, July 2014 (Page 3 of 4) PRIVACY NOTICE: See our privacy policy on www.usps.com.

Moving?

Make sure your subscription moves with you!

To notify us of your new address, find your **Clinics Account Number** (located on your mailing label above your name), and contact customer service at:

Email: journalscustomerservice-usa@elsevier.com

800-654-2452 (subscribers in the U.S. & Canada)
314-447-8871 (subscribers outside of the U.S. & Canada)

Fax number: 314-447-8029

Elsevier Health Sciences Division
Subscription Customer Service
3251 Riverport Lane
Maryland Heights, MO 63043

*To ensure uninterrupted delivery of your subscription, please notify us at least 4 weeks in advance of move.

Printed and bound by CPI Group (UK) Ltd, Croydon, CR0 4YY

03/10/2024

01040403-0011